Mediterranean Diet for Women

Definitive Guide to Hundreds of Quick, Delicious Recipes to Adapt Healthy Lifestyle

Vernon Potter

Text Copyright © Vernon Potter

Legal & Disclaimer

The information contained in this book and its contents is not designed to replace or take the place of any form of medical or professional advice; and is not meant to replace the need for independent medical, financial, legal or other professional advice or services, as may be required. The content and information in this book has been provided for educational and entertainment purposes only.

The content and information contained in this book has been compiled from sources deemed reliable, and it is accurate to the best of the Author's knowledge, information and belief. However, the Author cannot guarantee its accuracy and validity and cannot be held liable for any errors and/or omissions. Further, changes are periodically made to this book as and when needed. Where appropriate and/or necessary, you must consult a professional (including but not limited to your doctor, attorney, financial advisor or such other professional advisor) before using any of the suggested remedies, techniques, or information in this book.

Upon using the contents and information contained in this book, you agree to hold harmless the Author from and against any damages, costs, and expenses, including any legal fees potentially resulting from the application of any of the information provided by this book. This disclaimer applies to any loss, damages or injury caused by the use and application, whether directly or indirectly, of any advice or information presented, whether for breach of contract, tort, negligence, personal injury, criminal intent, or under any other cause of action.

You agree to accept all risks of using the information presented inside this book.

You agree that by continuing to read this book, where appropriate and/or necessary, you shall consult a professional (including but not limited to your doctor, attorney, or financial advisor or such other advisor as needed) before using any of the suggested remedies, techniques, or information in this book.

Table of Contents

Mediterranean Diet for Women

Introduction

7-Minute Workout for Seniors is a fitness book that specifically focuses on the benefits of exercise for seniors. The idea of this book is to provide information and inspiration to ensure that seniors can continue to live active, healthy lifestyles in old age. This book provides both a workout regime as well as advice on how to prepare for it. Because this book focuses on older individuals, it also includes some useful information about growing old, reminding readers that aging need not mean the end of physical activity and comfort with one's body.

This book has been written with the intention that it can be used by anyone, regardless of their educational background. It includes information on the importance of regular exercise for a healthy lifestyle and details of various exercises that can be carried out without any special equipment. These exercises are particularly geared towards individuals who may not have much strength or energy but with practice, can become more comfortable with their bodies and begin to move more independently. This book has been well-received by users because it does not require any sort of specific pre-existing condition in order to make use of its contents. It does not focus on fitness in terms of weight loss but rather, as a means to improve quality of life for older individuals. It has also been praised for its multiple useful tips which remind readers that the 7-minute workout is not just about getting fitter but also about being able to move more in general.

Chapter 1: The Benefits of Doing the 7-Minute Workout

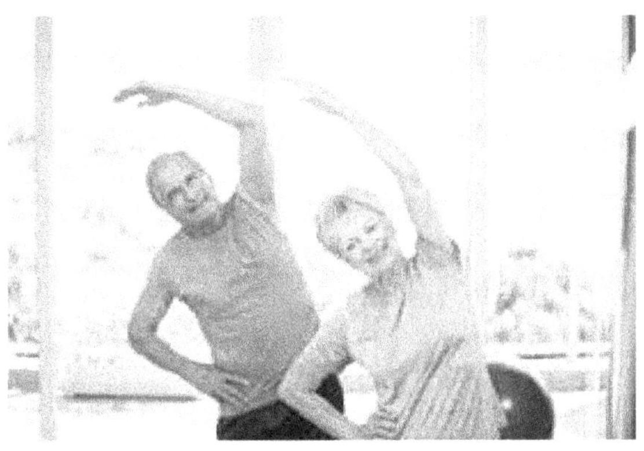

The 7-minute workout is beneficial in many ways.

The fact that the workout only takes seven minutes is great for working adults who do not have much time to work out but want to stay fit. This is also beneficial for children's after-school activities, as kids tend to be very busy and would not have the time nor patience to do a long workout. This is also beneficial because it requires only your body weight and no fancy equipment.

The 7-minute Workout could also be used to help individuals suffering from chronic diseases such as diabetes, hypertension, and heart disease by reducing their risk of developing certain diseases associated with sedentary lifestyles. It reduces the risk of developing other illnesses (e.g. obesity) that can lower your quality of life.

The 7-minute Workout is not just for adults; it is also beneficial to children and teens. It helps in fostering a healthy lifestyle early in life and ultimately lowering the risk of developing illnesses that are associated with sedentary lifestyles (e.g. heart disease, diabetes, obesity). Kids can do these exercises at home as often as possible because they only take seven minutes and they do not need expensive equipment.

The seven-minute workout is structured into four intervals. The workout has three different levels, each with their own workout routine.

I. Warm-up: Jumping jacks, High Knees, Butt Kicks and Star Jumps (each circuit for 30 seconds).

II. Strength Training: Squats (15 repetitions), Push-ups, Lunges (each circuit for 30 seconds). III. Core Strengthening: Crunches and Planks (each circuit for 30 seconds).

IV. Cool Down: Supermans and Back Extensions, Tricep Dips with a chair (each circuit for 30 seconds).

Benefits of doing the 7 minute workout to the old:

1) You will save yourself precious time in the mornings.

2) You will feel fresh and energized after your workout.

3) The workout is perfect for beginners.

4) It will help you build very lean muscle.

5) You can get very good results with this routine even if it is your first time working out.

6) It is a best way to maintain healthy weight.

7) It is an easy home workout, which requires just a pair of dumbbells, and a chin-up bar (or two chairs).

Gravity training utilizes the force of gravity as a resistance and does not require any special equipment or the purchase of expensive gym memberships.

Yoga is the practice of achieving physical, mental and spiritual balance through breathing, relaxation, and postures. Many people consider yoga as a way to reduce stress and improve overall health. Regular practice can be beneficial for flexibility, muscle strength, cardiovascular fitness, balance and coordination.

The 7-Minute Workout for Seniors has many benefits:

In order to improve performance in a physical activity it is necessary to do exercise. This does not mean that all exercise will increase performance in this activity it simply means it is necessary to do some exercise. Exercise can have many different benefits depending on the person's goals for their fitness program. In general exercise will strengthen our muscles and cardiovascular system which in turn will make us more fit. We often take for granted the many benefits we get from exercising. If you exercise regularly you will not only be healthier but happier as well. When we exercise our body releases endorphins which are said to make us feel good and happy. The endorphins also make us feel like having more energy too!

The 7-Minute Workout is said to be designed for seniors but can be beneficial to anyone who is a novice exerciser or has poor health, such as heart disease or diabetes. This workout consists of three rounds of seven exercises that should last about seven minutes in total. It is important to warm up before performing this workout and cool down after it as well. The author suggests that you should try to do this workout three times a week. The 7-Minute Workout for Seniors consists of 10 exercises. It takes only six minutes in total to do the circuit once. Perform one set of each exercise in the first minute and then one set of two exercises in the second minute, three sets of two exercises in the third minute and finally four complete rounds. These exercises are:

The core is a group of muscles that help stabilize your body during movement and keep it upright on both land and water. Strengthening your core muscles will help improve your performance in activities such as dancing, swimming, running or cycling. Core strengthening exercises usually target the lower back, upper back, abdominal muscles and hips.

The 7-Minute Workout for Seniors consists of three minutes of core exercises. The six exercises are:

The muscles in our body can be divided into two groups based on their location and function. Flexor muscles bend the joint and extensor muscles straighten it. There are some muscles that do both flexion and extension at the same time, such as the hip muscle. The 7-Minute Workout for Seniors consists of three minutes of strength exercises. These exercises target flexor and extensor muscles and help improve your performance in activities such as walking, running, swimming or golfing. The six exercises are:

The three strength training exercises are:

The last three minutes of this 7-minute workout is known as the cool-down and consists of three exercises. These exercises help relax your muscles after a hard workout :

These four sets together make up 6 minute circuit in a 7 minute workout. The book gives many reasons why we should exercise and participate in different physical activities such as dancing. The author states that one of the best ways to achieve a healthy body is by reducing our risk of developing many illnesses such as heart disease, obesity, diabetes, osteoporosis and depression. The author states that it is also important to eat a healthy diet because the food we eat can help our muscles recover faster after exercising or help them grow. The author also claims that by improving our health we can save money on medical bills and also have better quality of life.

The 7-Minute Workout for Seniors has proven to be beneficial throughout many stages of life, but particularly when beginning a fitness program or being diagnosed with heart disease or diabetes as stated in the introduction. This workout has also been proven to maintain muscle strength as we get older which is very important because it can improve balance and reduce the risk of falling which is one of the leading causes of death for seniors. This workout is also beneficial before and after a surgery. It can help with rehabilitation after the surgery and it will also help you get back into shape faster. This workout can improve cardiovascular fitness, balance, coordination, bone density and muscle strength. The 7-Minute Workout for Seniors is also beneficial for individuals who have chronic diseases such as diabetes, osteoporosis or heart disease because it can help reduce your risk of developing other diseases associated with sedentary lifestyles such as obesity or cardiovascular disease.

The 7-Minute Workout is designed to be done at home, but you can do this workout almost anywhere: at the gym, in your dorm room or in a hotel room. There are no special equipment needed to do this workout except for the following (if you don't have them at home) It is recommended that anyone who has just started exercising should begin by doing the exercises in the circuit three times and then working their way up to five times. It is also suggested that you progress from one circuit to another by increasing your repetitions (e.g., three sets of 10 each exercise). In order to improve your cardiovascular fitness you can do exercises such as jogging, walking, or cycling. Since you will be performing three circuits of this workout it is suggested that you perform the cardiovascular exercise for 10 minutes. The author suggests that for each circuit you should work up to about 80 percent of your maximum heart rate and then decrease it in order to recover. It is also suggested that the cool down should last about 1-2 minutes. It is also important that you drink plenty of water throughout each day and eat a healthy diet in order for your muscles to recover faster.

Chapter 2: How to do the 7-minute Workout

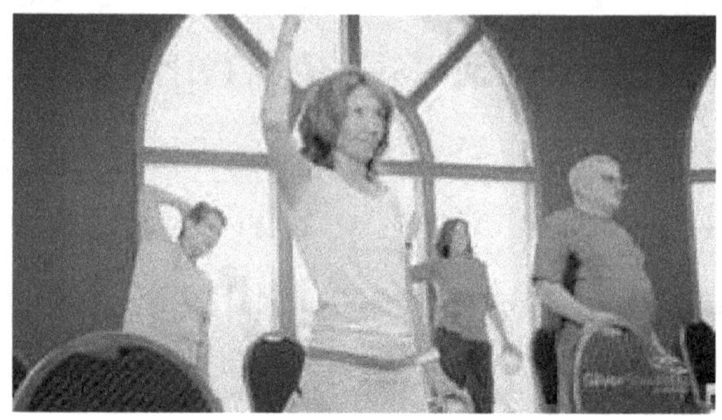

This introduces the reader to the different exercises that can be incorporated in the 7 Minute Workout. It describes a range of bodyweight exercises that can be carried out without any special equipment but with varying levels of intensity

For example:

1) Standard push-ups – performed on hands and toes on a hard surface such as a floor – can build strength, improve posture, and help prevent injuries. This is one of the most simple exercises that anyone can do anywhere at any time. This exercise can be

made harder by performing a push-up on one's knees instead of the standard position.

2) Squats – performed in a standing position with the feet at hip distance apart and then bending down until the knee is at right angles or close to it. This will help to build strength in the core and lower body, as well as improving overall balance.

3) Lunges – performed in a standing position with one foot forward and one back. As you lunge, focus on keeping your upper body straight and upright with your weight on the heel of your front foot. This will improve overall strength in the legs, improve balance, as well as working out different muscles depending on which leg is used during the lunge.

4) Planks – performed with the body in a straight line and supported on the hands and toes. This exercise is designed to

strengthen the core and increase overall flexibility.

5) Crunches – this exercise can be done by lying on your back with your knees bent and feet flat on the ground, or alternatively, for those who are more mobile, it can be preformed by sitting up with legs crossed to build strength in the core.

6) Raises – this is another simple abdominal exercise that anyone can do anywhere at any time. It involves simply drawing one's shoulders up towards their ears, holding for a few seconds and then lowering back down again.

This also focuses on the importance of exercise to the aging population, who are often perceived as a sedentary population who are not as active. However, close examination reveals that there is an active senior population in old age and it is important to recognise this and continue the activity into old age. Despite this, activity levels do start to fall off after around 65 years of age, so it is important for seniors to continue exercising despite many thinking that they don't need the exercise in their older age. This chapter also explains the difference between physical activity and exercise, with exercise referring to any intentional movement done with a specific goal.

The difference between physical activity and exercise are:

1) Physical activity is any activity done outside of work that requires energy to perform

2) Exercise is a physical activity that has a specific goal. E.g. running to lose weight, swimming to improve stroke technique

3) Physical activity can be unpaid e.g. gardening, walking with friends, walking to work

4) Exercise is paid for e.g. gym, swimming lessons, aerobics class

It gives a thorough overview of the benefits of physical activity for seniors and focuses on the importance of being active as part of a healthy lifestyle, through both exercise and daily activities. By giving examples it tries to raise awareness in people about the necessity of staying active as part of an overall healthy lifestyle and that growing old does not mean having to stop doing things one enjoys or is good for them in general.

If you're 60 or older, the thought of becoming frail, suffering injuries from falls, and losing your independence is often a real worry, even if it isn't already happening. Our body changes as we age —

and often in ways we don't like. We naturally lose 1-2 percent of our lean muscle mass every year after the age of 50. This gradual loss of muscle and strength is barely noticeable at first—until we wake up one day surprised that our physical ability is not what it used to be.

What if I could show you how to reverse muscle loss and reclaim your strength, balance, and energy faster than you ever thought possible?

It doesn't matter if you're 60 or 100 years old, or if you've been active or inactive your entire life. It doesn't matter if you're currently walking miles every day or struggling just to get up from a chair. It doesn't even matter if your health is perfect or imperfect. This book will show you how to transform your body and your life, no matter who you are, irrespective of your current state of health and fitness.

The book explains the core principle of the program: 'Use it or lose it'. It explains why this is fundamental to both staying healthy and preventing falls as you age. It presents the science behind how exercise can decline with old age and how exercise can prevent or at least minimise these declines. Furthermore, it gives examples of what exercises one can do as part of their program to combat these declines in physical abilities.

It discusses why balance is important for an active life and also goes through a number of ways one can improve their balance. It also has an entire chapter dedicated to the importance of staying physically fit in order to prevent falls. This chapter goes through what causes falls, common myths about preventing falls and the science behind why exercises can help you stay balanced. It also gives examples of exercises that can be used as part of your program and how often you should do them in order to stay balanced. During the last few years there has been an increasing body of research on the topic whether brain training programs designed to improve cognitive functions such as memory, attention and decision-making are effective and reliable. The term does not include persons administered anesthesia or other psychoactive drugs while they are in an operating room, recovery room, intensive care unit or any other environment related to the practice of surgery or medicine. The term neurocognitive aging is the same as normal age-related cognitive decline. The main difference is that normal age-related cognitive decline is more global and diffuse, whereas neurocognitive aging involves areas of the brain that are more or less impacted than others.

Neurocognitive decline does not include gradual change in personality over time which happens with normal aging called "normal personality reorganization". Consequently, neurocognitive decline can occur independent of personality changes. One distinctive aspect of neurocognitive aging is that it substantially interferes with the individual's ability to pursue meaningful and purposeful activities during middle and late adulthood. As a result, the process of aging often leads to considerable disability and dependency in individuals who are otherwise physically healthy. Neurocognitive decline is not a disease. It is simply a natural process that everyone experiences as they age.

According to the research conducted by Eyal Shahar and colleagues on elderly individuals who regularly spent time outdoors, cognitive functioning was observed to be greater in those individuals compared to those who did not spend as much time outdoors. This was connected to activity of the hippocampus, which is an area of the brain associated with spatial knowledge, memory, and emotion. Other research has found that when elderly patients who suffered from Alzheimer's were exposed to nature for two months they showed visible improvements in brain functioning. This included increases in activity of the hippocampus, cerebellum, and superior parietal lobule, which are areas of the brain associated with memory. Staying physically active is important for everyone, but it's especially vital for older adults who are more at risk of falling and having other injuries. This book provides a series of 12 exercises that can be done in just 7 minutes and that will increase strength, improve balance, build coordination, and more. Each exercise takes only a few minutes to learn. Already in the first week of doing the program you will be able to see great results in your body, and over time you will transform your fitness level and your confidence level!

Chapter 3: Three Powerful Techniques to Make Exercise a Habit

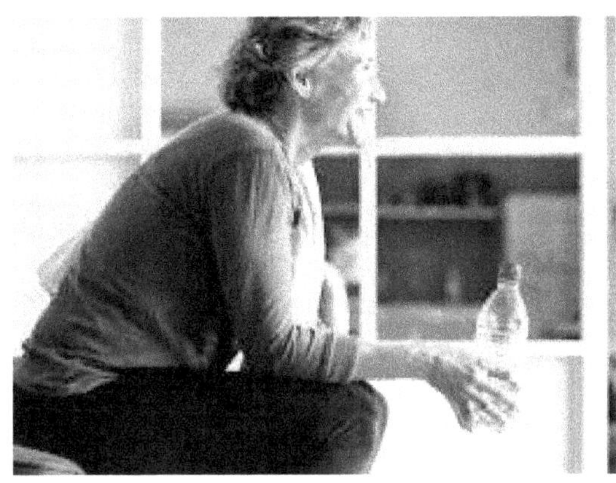

So you know from the previous 2 chapters that exercise is important and it will help you achieve your health, fitness and weight loss goals faster.

However, to make sure exercise becomes a habit, you need to use a specific approach. On this chapter I'll explain to you the 3 powerful techniques that will ensure your success. These techniques are: Decide what to exercise Focus on one thing at a time Implement the right rewards system

1. Decide What To Exercise This is so important! Don't just let yourself go or do what feels good at the moment. Instead, decide on the type of exercise program that you will do. For example, your goal is to lose weight, so instead of just running every day for 30 minutes, decide to do interval running. You may think interval training is just another way of exercising but it's not! If you want to gain more knowledge about interval training (and why I believe this type of training is the best) read Born To Run by Christopher McDougall. So "decide what to exercise" doesn't necessarily mean you need to get a gym membership or equipment (although those things can help). Even if there's no gym nearby or you are too busy, all you really need are your body and your mind.

2. Focus On One Thing At A Time Decide what to exercise. You have to decide

everything at once. So for example, if your goal is to lose weight and look better, decide that you will do the following: Interval running 3 times a week Weight training 3 times a week Yoga 1 time a week 15 minute meditation Daily water consumption of 2 liters Start with step 1! Don't worry about the others yet. It's important that you focus on only one thing at a time and when you've completed it, move on to the next one. So you may ask me: "How do I know which one to focus on first?" That's a great question. The answer is to ask yourself what's the most important for your situation. If you are overweight, it's very likely that exercise will help you burn more calories and thus lose more weight. So maybe put the interval running first and then move on to weight training later when you can fit it into your schedule. Decide what to exercise, this is half of the battle!

3. Implement The Right Rewards System

The best thing about having a goal (like losing weight) is not just reaching it but also achieving smaller rewards along the way. This will keep you motivated and push you to stick to your plan. You can also use these rewards to make yourself feel better about yourself! Here is a list of rewards that I recommend: Decide on the 1st reward you will give yourself (could be a new pair of workout shoes or a nice dinner) Make sure your rewards are limited (don't go overboard with them, choose something reasonable like two rewards for every 5 pounds) Find ways to enjoy these benefits, like eating a nice meal at the mall or window shopping

Now go out there and find a cool exercise program that's right for you. Make sure it's something you enjoy doing and can do regularly.

Technique 1: Habit Stacking

Habit stacking is a technique that will force you to do a series of habits. Our brain is lazy, which is good from one perspective, because once we've learned something it'll be easier for us to repeat it in the future. However, just like all other things, our brain needs some kind of stimulation so we stay on top of things. Habit stacking helps us with this by forcing us to initiate several habits at once and then take the actions needed to complete them.

One powerful application of habit stacking for exercise is a method called Run-Walk-Run .

What it is:

You alternate running with walking, so in other words you run and then walk. By doing this, you are able to exercise more efficiently and burn more calories.

How will this help me?

The answer to this question is really simple: if you walk more than you run, your heart rate and breathing will slow down instead of speeding up like when running. This means that your heart has to work less hard for the same amount of time. The result of this is that your body will burn fewer calories on a given period of time than if you were running all the time.

Technique 2: Conditioned Cues

This is an interesting technique that will allow you to prepare your mind for exercise and make it into a habit. It's very similar to how Pavlov's dog was conditioned to salivate in anticipation of food.

What is it?

You associate certain cues with exercising. For example, if you want to work out at the beach, then you may decide that when you start seeing the ocean, it's time for your run or walk workout. The idea is that once you start feeling that cue, your body (and your brain) will automatically prepare for exercise and you'll have a better chance of staying active throughout the day.

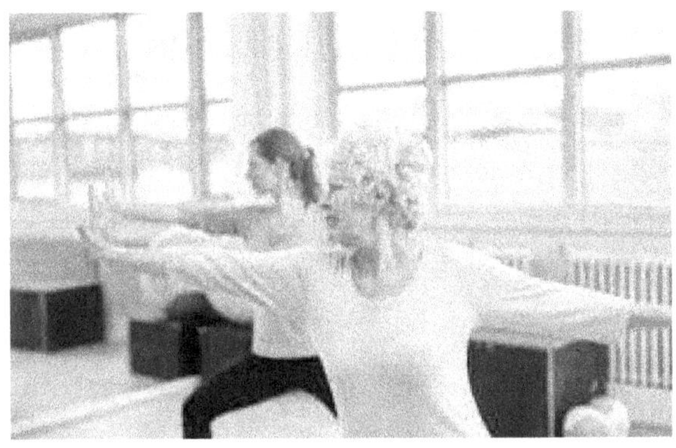

Technique 3: Intrinsic Reward Statements

This technique is somewhat similar to habit stacking but it's also a little bit different. The basic idea here is that you intersperse different activities into your workout. For example, instead of just running for 30 minutes, you can interleave jogging with jumping jacks. This will help you stay alert and active throughout the whole workout session.

Another example would be for weight training. Instead of just doing the same thing over and over again, you could do an exercise (like bench presses), then do something different (like bicep curls), then go back to bench presses and so on. This will keep your mind from getting bored and thus keep you more active throughout the workout session.

What is it:

This technique, pretty much like its name suggests, involves creating a visual representation of your exercise routine. This could be something like a poster with pictures to remind you of your workout plan for the week. Just seeing that reminder everyday can be enough to force you to act on it. Another option is to use an app or software program that helps you make the chart so you don't have to do the work yourself. There are two programs I really recommend: My Fitness Pal (fitnesspal.com) and Fitocracy (fitocracy.com).

How will it help me:

This technique is a bit different from the previous two. But personally I find it the most powerful of them all because you can use it no matter what your goal is. The idea behind this is that you create a goal and then you stick to it by posting it somewhere public where everybody can see. This way, if you don't start working towards your goal, people will notice and you'll feel bad about not taking action.Next time we'll be talking about how to make exercise a habit so stay tuned! In the meantime, keep on working out.

Key takeaways

Creating an exercise schedule that works best for you is not enough. That's why you need to learn how to make exercise a habit and start doing it without putting too much effort into it. I've outlined three techniques that will help you do just that:

1. Implementation Intentions

2. Habit Stacking

3. Visualization

There's one more technique you can use, which is a combination of the first two: First, make your schedule and then create an implementation intention to start implementing the schedule. This way you can make sure your schedule is not just sitting on a piece of paper but it's actually working for you.

Chapter 4: Great Results at Home with Little or No Equipment

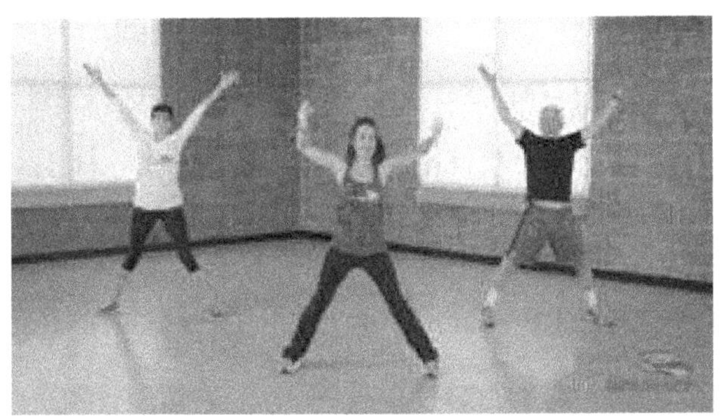

During the coronavirus pandemic, workout equipment flew off the shelves, with millions of people scrambling to put together a home gym because fitness centers were closing across the country. Equipment such as weights, exercise bikes, and rowers were out of stock for months. The good news is exercise can be just as effective without a gym or workout equipment. You can easily achieve the same results—or even better—exercising at home with little or no workout equipment using something called "functional training."

Functional Training

Functional training mimics activities or specific skills you perform at home, at work, or in sports to help you thrive in your daily life. This kind of training is effective because it uses different muscles simultaneously and also emphasizes core stability — the control of muscles around the abdomen and back that protect your spine when you move. For example, performing squats with a chair trains the same muscles you use when you rise from a chair, pick up an object from the ground, climb stairs, or hike up a mountain.

Many fitness and rehabilitation experts, including myself, have known for a while that functional training is the most effective way to train. Finally, the research is catching up with our observations. Functional training has now been shown in multiple studies to produce results that are superior to most other forms of exercise for diverse groups of people, including young military personnel, middle-aged females with low back pain, and (of course) older adults.14

One study demonstrated that high-intensity functional training was safe and effective for improving balance and independence in individuals aged 65 and older who had dementia and were living in nursing homes.15 Another showed that functional training significantly improved the golf swing and fitness level of golfers aged between 60 and 80 years old.16

By training your muscles to work functionally, you'll prepare your body to perform well in a variety of tasks that are important to your daily life—and you can do it at home with the aid of "equipment" readily available, such as a backpack filled with canned goods, to increase the difficulty level of exercise.

Exercising at Home

There are several additional benefits to exercising at home versus going to a gym:

•   The ease and convenience of exercising at home removes demotivating barriers. You don't have to drive to the gym, change your clothes in a room full of strangers, or wait for workout equipment to free up.

•   The gym can be an intimidating place for some older adults. But self-consciousness or fear of what others may think is not a concern with functional training at home.

•   For older adults who don't function well enough to leave home without assistance, going to the gym can be difficult or impossible. Exercising at home is the only way for these people to improve strength, balance, and function.

•   The price tag of a gym membership can be an obstacle for many older adults on fixed incomes. Cost is not an issue with workouts at home that require little or no equipment.

Combination Approach

The real secret to this program is the integration of higher-intensity training (discussed in the last chapter) and functional training, adapted for older adults. You won't find this combined approach to exercise for older adults in many other places, but it's a method that will allow you to safely and quickly achieve great results at home with little or no equipment.

You may be wondering at this stage why you couldn't just do something else that needs no equipment — such as walking — for exercise. It's certainly true that walking is another form of functional training that doesn't require equipment and can be good for your health, but in the next chapter I'll explain why walking alone isn't enough to reverse age-related muscle loss.

Key Takeaways

• You can easily achieve the same or even better results exercising at home with little or no workout equipment using "functional training."

• Multiple studies have shown functional training to produce results that are superior to most other forms of exercise for diverse groups of people, including older adults.

• The real secret to this program is the integration of higher-intensity training with functional training adapted for older adults.

It will allow you to safely and quickly achieve great results at home with little or no equipment.

Action Steps

•   Prepare yourself for exercising at home by making sure you have the following items handy:

o   A backpack filled with heavy items (such as canned goods) for resistance.

o   A pair of five-pound ankle weights.

•   If you're a family member or a caregiver for an older adult you'd like to help with exercise, prepare them for exercising at home by making these items available.

•   Only use a pair of five-pound ankle weights, and not heavier ones, when you exercise.   Lighter   weights   are   more comfortable and will allow you to perform the exercises with better form.

It is important to note that the risk of a heart attack or stroke is highest in the first three days following a sudden change in physical activity levels. Therefore, it is critical to speak with your doctor before starting an exercise program.

•   It's best to begin with about 3 minutes of exercise per session and build up gradually over the next few weeks to as much as 10 minutes at a time.

•   It's not necessary to do all twelve exercises every week — in fact, you may find that you feel more comfortable adding just two or three new exercises each week.

•   Workout every day at home (ideally) or 3 days/week for optimal results from this program.

- It is important to incorporate a warm-up and a cool-down into your home workout to prevent injury and experience greater benefits.

- Perform each exercise with perfect form at least two or three times before moving on to the next exercise.

- Check with your doctor before starting this program.

- To maintain gains obtained from working out, it's vitally important to resist the urge to take breaks when you can easily fit in a workout routine.

What you need to know about training at home:

- It's common, especially in older adults, to experience some aches and pains after a workout. If this occurs, stick with the program, but cut back on the intensity of the exercise or change the duration of your workout until you can tolerate it well. For example, instead of doing 10 minutes of walking, do 5 minutes walking and 5 minutes of easy stretching.

• If you experience chest pain that is not relieved by medicine or does not go away within a few minutes after stopping exercise, it may be a sign of unstable angina (a warning sign for heart attack). Seek medical help right away.

• If you experience tightness, pain, or numbness in the area of your chest that does not subside within a few minutes, it may be a sign of a heart attack that is occurring right now. Seek medical help right away as this can cause sudden death.

• If you experience sudden dizziness or nausea while exercising and it does not go away within a few minutes after stopping exercise, it may be a sign of an inner ear disturbance—a warning sign for stroke. Seek medical help right away.

• If you have high blood pressure or a history of heart attack or stroke, consult with your doctor about starting this program slowly with lower-intensity exercise and shorter duration at first. I recommend that these individuals start by doing 3 minutes/day of exercise and progress gradually by adding 1 minute of exercise each week. When they can tolerate 10 minutes per day, they can return to the regular program.

• If you have osteoporosis, a history of broken bones, or if you have ever fainted due to low blood pressure, it is very important to talk to your doctor about having an exercise stress test before starting this program. Most individuals older than 60 who have had heart attacks or strokes should also have an exercise stress test.

• Seek a doctor's advice if you have had any of the following conditions and are considering starting this program: hypertension, heart condition (including an irregular heart beat), diabetes, chronic lung disease, joint problems, or smoking.

• If there is any doubt about your ability to exercise—due to health problems or medications you are taking—you should consult with your doctor before starting this program.

Chapter 5: The 7 Minute Workout for Seniors: Rest and Recovery

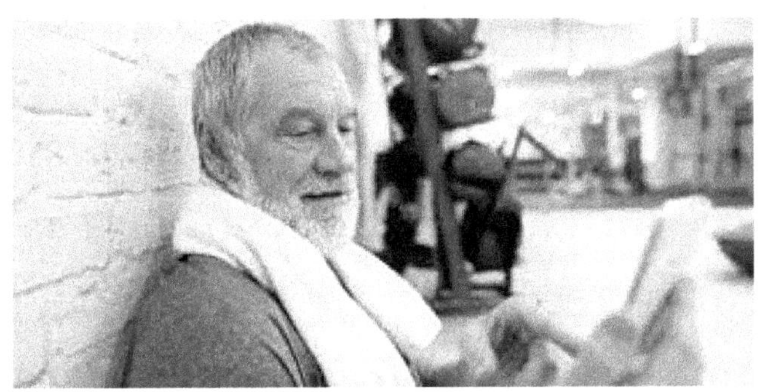

This chapter focuses on the rest and recovery aspect of the 7-Minute Workout. The author explains that using the seven minutes to work out is not enough and that a routine such as this must be complemented by adequate time spent in rest and recovery. The rest and recovery aspect of the 7-Minute Workout is made up of three phases: Early Recovery, Late Recovery and Active Recovery.

Early Recovery phase

In the Early Recovery phase, the author recommends that you should get off of the floor or out of the water and sit for a short period of time. Here you can even perform some gentle stretching if this is comfortable. If you exercise in a pool or at the beach, then you can simply stay in the water and float on your back for a few minutes. In this phase, it is recommended that you refrain from any intense exercises. It is said to be important to separate this from the Early Recovery phase and perform it about twenty minutes after the workout is completed.

While moving into the Late Recovery phase, it is recommended that you perform energizing exercises such as arm circles or leg swings. This should be done for approximately 2-3 minutes after the workout has ended. It is also recommended that you continue your rest and try not to sit or lay down for long periods of time. The author suggests that you may want to begin performing gentle stretching at this point but stay away from Yoga or Pilates because they increase flexibility which can cause an imbalance in your muscles and joints. The Late Recovery phase should last about five minutes.

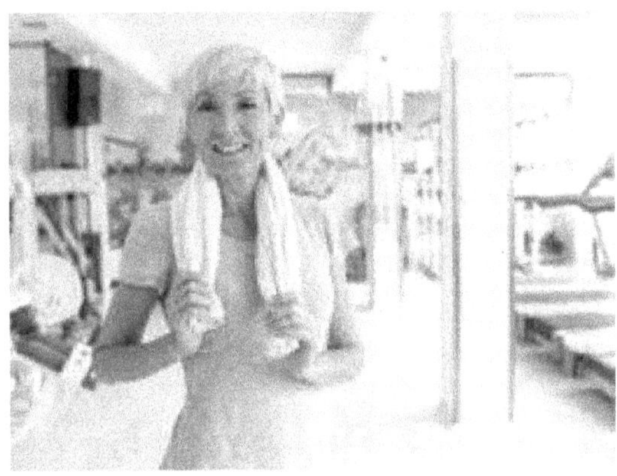

The Late Recovery phase

This is the most important phase of rest and recovery because this is when your body becomes ready for its next major stress or challenge. The author explains that we are not at a state where we need to be worrying about recovering our bodies in this case as we already have. It is said that during this time it can be important to get sufficient amounts of sleep because during sleep our body heals itself with increased blood flow. During sleep the blood flow to our brain increases by 50% and we achieve REM sleep in which our concentration levels are better and the brain consolidates memories.

Active Recovery,

This period of training is low intensity and consists mainly of aerobic activity such as walking or cycling to improve circulation around the body. The author explains that this should be done for 30–60 minutes. This helps return blood that has built up in our muscles after exercise back into the blood stream. If Active Recovery Phase is not followed, there is a danger of overtraining because after several days of hard training you will have fatigue which could lead to illness, injury or burnout.

When your muscles and joints are in the Early Recovery phase, you can try to strengthen your connective tissues with exercises such as yoga. By doing this the author says you can improve flexibility and prevent injury which could otherwise be caused by a weak or brittle muscle. The author states that performing yoga for a short 3 minutes after a Workout is enough to significantly increase circulation, heart rate and respiration which will enhance recovery in addition to reducing stress and anxiety.

The second half of this chapter provides many different methods of how you can improve rest and recovery such as stretching, self massage, tapping and meditation. The final section of this chapter is titled "Yoga, Strengthening and Balance." The author explains how the practice of yoga (see Yoga) has proven to be beneficial for all ages. The author then explains how yoga can be incorporated into a 20 or 30-minute workout because we are all short on time and this is the main reason why the 7-Minute Workout for Seniors was invented in the first place.

The author explains that a good warm up should last 10–20 minutes and can include exercises such as walking, jogging, cycling, swimming or any other activity that gets your heart rate up. After this the author says that we should do a circuit of exercises for 7 minutes. The 7-Minute Workout for Seniors consists of 10 exercises that should be performed in a circuit style. In the first minute perform 1 set of each exercise and then in the second minute perform 2 sets, and so on until you reach 7 sets. The author states that it is possible to perform this workout in both a fasted state or after eating. The author then provides a table with each exercise listed along with the page number where it can be found and details about how much weight to use/how deep to go and also which muscles that exercise works out. The circuit consists of the following exercises:

The last exercise in this circuit is a plank. The author states that the plank is a good way to measure progress because it has no weight requirement and only takes ten seconds to complete. The author says that when you begin the 7-Minute Workout for Seniors this plank should be held for 15–20 seconds and you should work towards increasing it to 60–90 seconds. This second half of this chapter contains information about Yoga, Strengthening and Balance. The author explains how by practicing yoga you can strengthen your muscles, improve balance, relieve stress and have more energy at rest. The author also claims that practicing yoga will improve your flexibility. The chapter starts off with a description of Yoga. The author then explains how yoga can be incorporated into a 20 or 30-minute workout and how to do each movement correctly. The following yoga postures are described with pictures to help you see the correct form:

Next are all the exercises that you can use if you are not doing a yoga routine such as squats, lunges, push-ups, bridges, calf raises and planks. These exercises will help strengthen the muscles and increase bone density in your body. You can do this along with walking or any other aerobic activity because it is said that "muscle strengthening is key to improving muscular health. Strength training has been linked to delaying the onset of physical disabilities, which reduces the risk of falling and fracturing bones." The last section in this chapter is for Balance Exercises. The author then explains how "improving our balance can reduce our risk of falling, which is important as falls are one of the leading causes of injuries and death among older adults." By doing these exercises you will be able to get your muscles ready for challenging movements that you will perform if you take dance lessons or go hiking with friends.

Chapter 6: Tips for Family Members and Caregivers

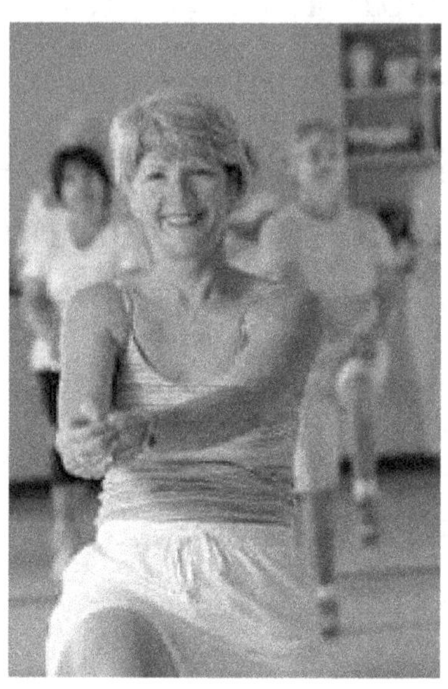

Older adults with memory issues or who lack the motivation to exercise will need help from another person.

Although we never want to force someone to exercise when they don't want to, persuasion is sometimes necessary because a persistent lack of movement leads to serious issues, such as debility, bed sores, and injuries from falls.

Older adults with memory issues or who lack motivation may have a difficult time starting and sticking with an exercise program. But I've found it becomes less challenging once exercise becomes routine, and changes in strength, balance, and energy become apparent after a few weeks.

The key to persuasion is a simple process I've created called the four Es: enthusiasm, empathy, encouragement, and ease. This process takes only a few minutes and has been effective with even my most exercise-resistant clients. Let's explore each step in detail.

Enthusiasm

Richard Simmons, the semi-retired American fitness instructor known for his eccentric and energetic personality, is a great example of enthusiasm at its best. It's difficult not to feel pumped up and motivated to move when you watch him.

So the first step in motivating someone is to be enthusiastic. Your enthusiasm is contagious, and it can shift another person's energy level and desire to exercise in powerful ways. To make enthusiasm work, you have to authentically feel it and express it in your words and body language.

Try to authentically feel and express enthusiasm in your voice, posture, gesture, and facial expression while saying something like, "Dad, it's time to exercise. It'll only take six minutes, and you'll feel great afterward. Let's do it!" If you encounter any resistance, move to the next step.

Empathy

The second step is to feel and express empathy: the ability to understand and share the feelings of another. It's important because a person is more likely to be open to your suggestions when they know you've understood and considered their perspective.

So to feel empathetic, you should know the common reasons why an older adult may not want to exercise: They may have lost hope that things will ever get better. They may be fearful that the aches and pains they experience daily will get worse if they exercise. They may feel constantly exhausted and don't know if they have the energy needed to exercise.

Whatever the reason, start by stepping into their shoes and feel what they may be feeling. Then express your understanding through your words and body language. Try to authentically feel and express empathy in your voice, posture, gesture, and facial expression while saying something like, "Dad, I can understand that you're feeling exhausted, and the aches that come with your age don't help. I also wonder if you've lost some hope that things can get better." It helps to pause for several seconds at this point to tune in to feelings that may be coming up for you and the other person. Then, move to the next step, which is to encourage the person.

Encourage

After feeling and expressing empathy, it's time to encourage the person to exercise.

For this to be effective, I suggest doing two things. First, understand the person's personal values and bring them into this step. A person's values can be things like determination or hope or respecting authority figures such as doctors. Second, remind the person of the benefits of exercise that are important to them. These benefits can be things like feeling more energized after exercising, gaining the ability to live more independently, feeling happier because they can avoid hospitalizations, or having more energy playing with the grandchildren.

Whatever the reason for exercising, keep it positive, and express it with passion in your words and body language.

Use this step to authentically feel and express passion in your voice, posture, gesture, and facial expression while saying something like, "Dad, you always told us growing up that sometimes things will get worse before they get better, and having hope will get you through these times. It's no different getting your body working better through exercise. Remember how much you want to get back to gardening? What do you say?" If the person still isn't convinced to exercise at this point, it's time for the final step.

Ease

The fourth and final step is to ease into exercise. Use this when the previous steps haven't persuaded the person to take action. Your goal is to make exercise something the person can try for a few repetitions to see how it feels, knowing they can stop any time.

To make this step work, I recommend you first openly acknowledge that the person really doesn't want to exercise. Then suggest that they try just a few repetitions of one exercise to see how it feels. Tell them they can stop any time.

Perform this step with enthusiasm, and encourage the person to continue exercising after they've started. With enthusiastic encouragement, most people won't stop exercising once they've begun and may even surprise you with their new motivation.

Use this step to authentically feel and express enthusiasm in your voice, posture, gesture, and facial expression while saying something like, "I totally understand that the idea of exercise doesn't sit well with you right now, but let's just do five chair squats and see how it feels. I'll help you, and you can stop any time if you don't want to continue after that. Come on, let's start now."

As the person approaches the fifth repetition of the exercise, enthusiastically encourage them to continue by saying something like, "Wow, you're looking really strong! I'm amazed by how well you're doing! Keep going, I know you've got it in you!"

Applying the four Es takes only a few minutes and has been effective with even my most exercise-resistant clients.

However, at times, nothing you do will persuade someone to exercise. It's best to yield to the person's wishes in these moments.

Fortunately, just two or three good workout sessions a week is enough to see improvements with this program in most adults. That may be all you will get out of someone who really doesn't like to exercise—but after a few weeks, they may be more motivated after noticing improvements in their strength, balance, and energy. So stay positive and be patient.

Key Takeaways

- The four Es can help persuade the person to exercise: enthusiasm, empathy, encouragement, and ease.

- The first step is to be enthusiastic. Your enthusiasm is contagious, and it can increase another person's desire to exercise. To make enthusiasm work, you have to authentically feel it and express it in your words and body language.

- The second step is to feel and express empathy: the ability to understand and share the feelings of another. A person is more likely to be open to your suggestions when they know you've understood and considered their perspective.

- The third step is to encourage. Understand the person's values and include them in your conversation, and remind them of the benefits of exercise that are important to them.

- The fourth and final step is to ease into exercise. Use this strategy when the previous steps haven't persuaded the person to exercise. The goal is to make exercise something the person can try for a few repetitions to see how it feels, knowing they can stop any time.

Action Steps

- If you're a family member or a caregiver for an older adult you'd like to help with exercise, practice the four Es a few times on your own to get comfortable with the method before using it to persuade them to exercise

Chapter 7: The Workout Routine

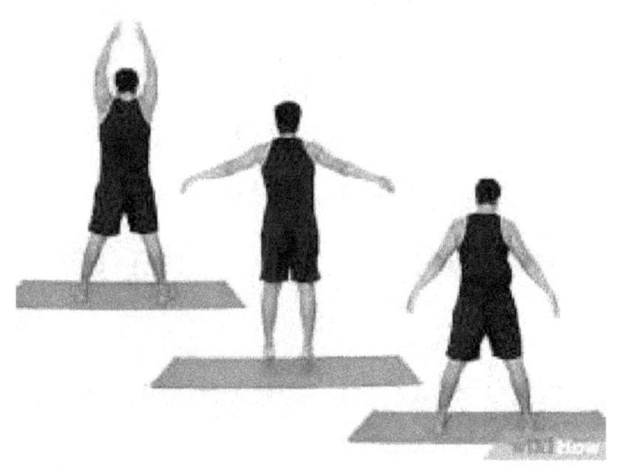

In this section, the exercise moves laid out in the previous chapter will be put together for a routine that will be suited to your fitness level. Determine your fitness level and take the fitness test in Chapter 4. Doctors recommend having at least 150 minutes of physical activity a week. Spread out over the week, that's 30 minutes of activity for five days. Workouts are great but you'll have to give your body time to adjust and recover. Two days of rest and recovery can be inserted midweek or during weekends. From 150 minutes, you'll build up to 225 minutes, and eventually 300 or more minutes a week. These routines aren't set in stone. As you progress and learn, and get used to the exertion, you'll have the confidence and the personal knowledge to mix and match exercise moves you feel would best suit your body's strength and endurance levels.

The plan is to do each level consistently for four weeks until you've increased your stamina and endurance, and could do more reps, more sets for longer periods. Before starting on any fitness routine, make sure that you've assessed your health and fitness functionality with the tests in Chapter 4. If you fall within the below average range, you'll start at the beginner level with a focus on 70% cardio to improve your stamina and 30% strength training. If you've an intermediate level result, the ratio is 60% cardio and 40% strength training. For those with results in the expert level, it'll be equal parts cardio and strength training. The routines outlined here are also adaptable to where you're most comfortable doing your exercises. A fifth of the exercises could be done outdoors - walking, cycling, and swimming. The rest can be done at home or at the gym. The exercise equipment needed is also minimal or easily adaptable with items readily found at home.

Work needs to be done to develop mobility and stamina if your fitness test shows below average results. Perform 15 minutes of stretching exercises to improve mobility and 15 minutes of simple cardio workouts.

Here's a sample stretching, strengthening, and cardio routine.

3 minutes of warm-up stretches

- Perform 2 times, Upper Back Stretch
- Perform 2 times, Chest Stretch

- Perform once on either side of the neck, Neck Stretch

- Perform 2 times, Sit and Reach Stretch

- Perform once for each leg, Inner Thigh Stretch

- Do 1 set of 16 reps, Shoulder Circles

- Do 1 set Hand Stretches

8 minutes of muscle strengthening & balance exercise

DAY 1

- 2 sets of 10 reps for each leg, Side Leg Raise

- 2 sets of 16 reps, Seated Shin Strengtheners

- 2 sets of 8 reps, Pliés

- 2 sets of 10 to 15 reps, Front Arm Raise

- 2 sets of 5 reps for each side, Side Bends

- 2 sets of 8 reps, Tummy Twists

- 2 sets of 10 reps for each leg, Knee Extensions

- 2 sets of 10 reps for each hand, Wrist Curls

- 4 sets of 15-20 steps, Toe the Line

- 2 sets of 10-second Flamingo Stands for each leg

- Perform 3 Clock Reaches for each side

DAY 2

- 2 sets of 10-second Flamingo Stands for each leg

- 2 sets of 10 reps, Side Leg Raise

- 2 sets of 10 to 15 reps, Front Arm Raises

- 2 sets of 5 reps for each side, Side Bends

- 2 sets of 8 reps, Tummy Twists

- 2 sets of 10 reps for each hand, Wrist Curls

- 2 sets of 10 to 12 reps, Bicep Curls
- 2 sets of 16 reps, Seated Shin Strengtheners
- 2 sets of 8 reps, Pliés
- 2 sets of 10 to 15 reps, Wall Push-Ups
- 2 sets of 10 reps for each leg, Knee Extensions

DAY 3

- 2 sets of 5 reps for each leg, Leg Lifts
- 2 sets of 15 reps, Seated Knee Lifts
- 2 sets of 10 reps, Knee Extensions
- 2 sets of 10 to 15 reps, Front Arm Raises
- 2 sets of 10 reps for each hand, Wrist Curls
- 2 sets of 10 to 12 reps, Bicep Curls
- 2 sets of 16-second Single Limb Stance with Arm for each leg
- Perform 3 Clock Reaches for each side

- 2 sets of 8 to 10 reps, Modified Burpees
- 2 sets of 5 reps for each side, Side Bends
- 2 sets of 15 reps, Seated Twists

DAY 4

- 2 sets of 5 reps for each leg, Leg Lifts
- Perform Bicycles for 30 seconds, rest, then go another 30 seconds
- 4 sets of 15-20 steps, Toe the Line
- Do 2 turns on the Speed & Agility Drill ladder
- 2 sets of 10 reps for each hand, Wrist Curls
- 1 set of 10 reps, Dumbbell Upright Row
- 2 sets of 10 to 15 reps, Wall Push-Ups
- Perform 3 Clock Reaches for each side
- 2 sets of 8 to 10 reps, Modified Burpees
- 2 sets of 8 reps, Pliés

- 2 sets of 16 reps, Seated Shin Strengtheners

DAY 5

- 2 sets of 10-second Flamingo Stands for each leg

- 2 sets of 16-second for each leg, Single Limb Stance with Arm

- 2 sets of 16 reps, Seated Shin Strengtheners

- 2 sets of 10 reps for each leg, Side Leg Raises

- 2 sets of 8 reps, Pliés

- 2 sets of 5 reps for each side, Side Bends

- 2 sets of 8 reps, Tummy Twists

- 2 sets of 15 reps, Seated Twists

- 1 set of 10 reps, Dumbbell Upright Row

- 2 sets of 10 to 15 reps, Wall Push-Ups

- 2 sets of 8 to 10 reps, Modified Burpees

15 minutes of cardio exercises

- 5 minutes marching in place

- 10 minutes of brisk walking

ALTERNATE CARDIO A

- a 15-minute bike ride or

ALTERNATE CARDIO B

- 5 minutes easy resistance on a stationary or elliptical bike

- 10 minutes medium resistance on a stationary or elliptical bike

2 minutes of cool down stretches

- Perform 2 times, Upper Back Stretch

- Perform 2 times, Chest Stretch

- Perform the cool down routine below:

1. March in place for 30 seconds.
2. Step your right foot forward to a lunge position and rest your hands on the middle part of your right thigh. Lunge forward taking caren't to let your knee go over your toes.

3. You should feel a bit of a stretch on your left calf. Hold the position for 16 counts. Switch positions and repeat step number 2 with your left leg.
4. Step your right foot behind and rest your hands on your hands on your right knee. Slowly bend from the waist pushing your buttocks backward and up.
5. You should feel a bit of a stretch on the back of your left thigh muscles. Hold the position for 16 counts. Switch positions and repeat step number 4 with your left leg.
6. March in place for 60 seconds. Stand with a wide stance and spread your arms upwards to stretch. Sweep your arms down to the side and raise them up again. Repeat this move for 8 counts.

Chapter 8: Is There an Ideal Diet?

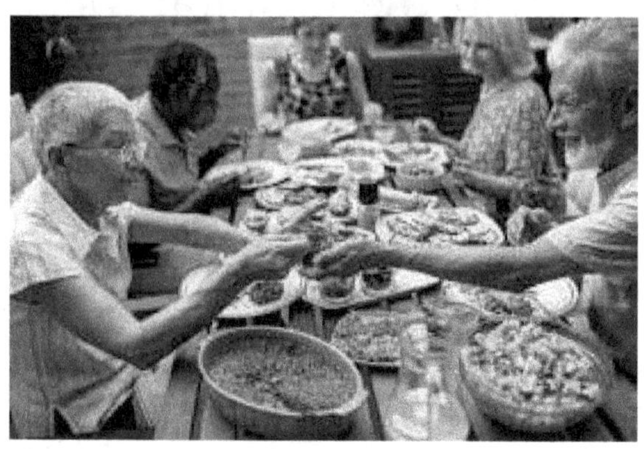

Walk into a bookstore and look for the section for books on diet. You will need time just to read the titles because the number of diets that are recommended is extensive. There are several reasons for this:

➢ Many people need help and guidance on weight loss and for managing conditions and illnesses: diabetes, heart disease, hypertension, cancers, immune disorders, and psychological problems among others.

➢ There is generally a belief that there is a magic diet, a silver bullet solution to lose weight, build muscle, cure disease, and live longer.

➤ Diet is all about eating, and people generally take eating very seriously as evidenced by the size of the cookbook section at the bookstore.

Let's take a quick look at some of the diets that are popular today, but with the understanding that while there are responsible ways to help with weight control and prevent or alleviate certain diseases, there is no single amazing diet that is the solution for everyone's problems. There is no "one size fits all" die because each of us has our own unique physiology, our own metabolic rate, our own sensitivities.

Popular Diets

Fasting has emerged recently as a way to health, happiness and a longer life, but you need to know that while the research involving worms and mice has been encouraging, the studies involving humans are mostly in the early stages. The more common approaches are intermittent fasting, conducted on a daily, repeating basis, such as the 16:8 fasting diet, which allows eating during an eight-hour period (e.g., 8 a.m. to 4 p.m.), and nothing to eat for the next 16 hours (4 p.m. to 8 a.m.). There are stricter versions, like 18:6. Alternatively, some try prolonged fasting, going for 24- or even 48- hour fasts, followed by a day of unlimited eating. People who practice this tend not to overeat on the non-fast days because their stomachs shrink a bit during the fast period,

➢ As a weightlifter seeking to build muscles, fasting diets are not advised for you.

Paleo diets harken back to paleolithic, simpler times when our distant ancestors were hunter-gatherers and ate "off the land," which means whatever they could find. This inspires diets today that avoid all refined and processed foods (which is commendable) and based on foods that our bodies evolved over millions of years to digest effectively.

A paleo diet limits foods like dairy products, grains and legumes, and potatoes that became available when farming and agriculture started around 10,000 years ago. Added salt is also avoided. Overall, the paleo diet is acknowledged as healthy and wholesome as long as the ratios of macronutrients are respected, and a diversity of foods is included so that adequate amounts of vitamins and minerals are included.

Keto diet, short for ketogenic, has a very specific objective: rapid weight loss through stimulation of fat burning. This is achieved by following a very high-fat, very low-carbohydrate diet, essentially replacing the carbs with fats. This results in a metabolic condition called ketosis, which is highly efficient in using stored and dietary fat, instead of carbs and stored glycogen, for energy. You burn fat; you lose weight. Another quality is the conversion of fat stored in the liver to ketones, which supply energy to the brain. Also, the keto diet has been shown to lower blood sugar and insulin levels, which may contribute to the prevention or reduction of diabetes and other disorders. Other benefits are a feeling of fullness (satiety) that reduces cravings to eat or snack and improved mood. Studies of the longer-term effects of keto and other very low-carb diets are underway.

While the keto diet appears to be effective for weight loss, it may not include sufficient protein for building muscle mass; at least 30 percent of your diet should be protein.

Mediterranean diet. Let's conclude with a diet that is not only gaining broad acceptance, but it is the closest to the ideal diet everyone is searching for. It includes a wide range of wholesome and great-tasting foods, is affordable, is credited by the medical community as being heart-healthy, and may help slow the onset of many other diseases, from diabetes to cancer.

This diet is based on the practices of long-term residents of the Mediterranean Basin, including parts of Italy, Spain, and France, who tend to live healthier, longer lives. But importantly, these people practice a lifestyle that includes not only diet, but also being physically active all their lives, keeping their weight at normal levels, and having a positive attitude towards life.

The components of the Mediterranean diet:

➢ A variety of fresh vegetables, fresh and dried fruits, nuts, and seeds, whole grains and cereals, fish, lean meat in small servings (e.g., six ounces), moderate quantities of dairy (mostly as cheese), eggs, extra virgin olive oil, and wine, mostly red, consumed in moderation.

Whatever diet you choose, remember that as a weightlifter and builder of strength and muscle, you need sufficient protein in your diet, and you should select foods that are low in saturated fats. Avoid salty, processed foods, fried foods, and anything containing large amounts of sugar. The next section details the good and bad sources of foods.

Food Sources: Good and Bad

The types and sources of the three macronutrients have been discussed in detail, but to summarize, here is a quick checklist of the good and the bad. While this chapter has been devoted to helping you to understand the foods that are most beneficial to your health and to improve your level of physical fitness, build muscle and make you stronger, there are sources of carbohydrates, proteins, and fat that you should avoid. To help your dietary planning, we've listed both the recommended sources of your macronutrients and the foods that have been designated as undesirable and potentially harmful.

According to nutritionists at MD Anderson Cancer Center:

Recommended carbohydrates sources include:

➢ Dairy products, including milk, yogurt, and cottage cheese, but with a preference for low-fat or non-fat since full-fat dairy products are high in saturated fats and calories. Non-dairy substitutes made from soy, almonds, and oats are also good sources of carbs. Dairy products also provide high-quality complete protein.

➢ Vegetables, which can be eaten without limitation since they are low in calories and rich in vitamins and minerals. Select a variety of colors (green, yellow, red, purple) which will provide a diversity of micronutrients.

➢ Fruits are high in natural sugars (which is why they taste sweet) and micronutrients. Fruit should be eaten without added sugar and in natural, solid form to preserve pulp, which adds valuable fiber. Many juices have added sugar and the pulp has been removed.

➢   Beans, peas, and lentils, known as legumes, provide high levels of carbohydrates, plus fiber and many of the 20 amino acids that comprise protein.

➢   Whole grains, including whole wheat, rye, buckwheat, spelt, corn, and oats, are high in carbs and are excellent sources of vitamin B and fiber. Refined grains do not have these added qualities.

Carbohydrate sources to avoid:

➢   Refined flours and sugar, found in crackers, most breads, cookies, breakfast cereals, and sugar, in most fruit juices, soft drinks, most athletic performance beverages, and candy.

Recommended protein sources include:

➢   Beans, including black, pinto, and kidney beans, plus lentils and soy products. Except for soy, the proteins are incomplete and need supplementation with grains and cereals.

➢   Nuts and seeds, including nut butters (sugar-free versions).

➢   Whole grains, including quinoa, rye, wheat, spelt, corn, and soy, with the caveat that the amino acids do not comprise complete protein.

➢   Animal protein from meat, poultry, fish and seafood, dairy, and eggs.

Protein sources to avoid:

➢   Processed meats, like sausages, salami, bacon, frankfurters (hot dogs), and canned lunch meats.

➢   Consumption of lean red meats should be limited to 18 ounces per week.

Recommended fat sources include:

➢   Vegetable oils, especially extra virgin olive oil, avocado oil, and canola oil, and secondarily, oils from corn, sunflower, and safflower.

➢   Fatty fish, notably coldwater salmon, tuna, mackerel, and sardines.

➢   Flax seeds, chia seeds, avocados, and olives.

➢   Nuts and seeds, and again, natural nut butters, no sugar added.

Fat sources to avoid:

➢   Fried foods, which are made with refined flour and absorb large amounts of oils that contain trans fats.

➢   Animal sources, including full-fat dairy like milk, butter, yogurt, cream cheese, and the fats on meats and poultry.

➢   Vegetable oils from coconut and palm sources, shortening (used in baking), soft tub margarines, and most packaged baked goods (read the labels for fat content).

Now, on to Chapter 7 and dismissing some common misconceptions about working out, getting into shape, building muscles, and gaining strength when you are 60-plus.

Chapter 9: Motivation and Commitment

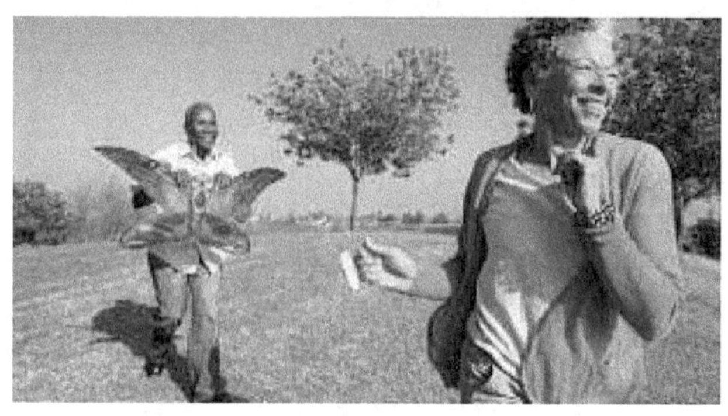

An important part of your long-term muscle and strength-building program is mental. Of course, it will be the weights, the reps, the sets, and the rests in between that will give you the lean muscle mass you want, but your state of mind will determine if you actually get started and if you will go the distance for the months and years of exercise it will take. Rome wasn't built in a day, and your impressive physique won't happen immediately.

The Motivation

In the initial chapter and at other points in this book, the importance of motivation was established as an incentive to getting your weightlifting and fitness program underway. No one can make you get into a regular, well-planned weightlifting program; you have to have the resolve and enthusiasm to take charge of your body, your health, and your appearance:

➤ If you have read this far, chances are good that you get it, "you're in."

➤ You imagine yourself lifting the barbells and dumbbells, doing the push-ups and pull-ups, the planks, the squats, and the splits.

➤ You feel committed to cardiovascular conditioning to help melt the extra pounds while you invest in your health and longevity.

➤ You feel better looking in the mirror in anticipation of the bigger, defined muscles you are going to build.

The Commitment

But will you have the determination and discipline to go the distance, to continue regularly with your bodybuilding and strengthening practices? Motivation is important at the beginning, but you need to have the discipline to stick to the routine even on days when you just don't have the drive, when you say, "I'll do it tomorrow."

You need to transcend the forces that hold you back, to break free of the constraints, and be committed no matter how tired or uninspired you are at that moment. Only then can you keep on track to meet your fitness and strengthening goals.

Commitment to succeed as a weightlifter, who builds muscle, who loses fat and excess weight, starts in the mind, which is the most effective and persuasive tool that will help you achieve your bodybuilding objectives. A positive attitude and the determination to work through the toughest movements will carry you through the worst of it with grit. Those who fail to make it, who give up, who quit, may be tough physically but don't have the mental toughness. Remember that your body will follow your mind.

Successful weightlifters at every level of training have developed positive thoughts to get themselves to the gym, to pick up the first weight of the session, to get through it with a full effort, no matter how tired or busy they were. You can adopt these thoughts, make them yours, let them carry you to the workout, and through the work, every time.

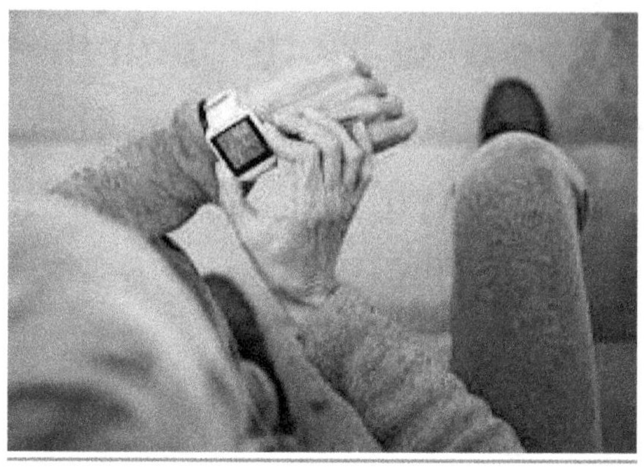

Positive Reinforcements

1. I'll just do a half-workout today, take it easy.

This works when you're tired and helps to get you started. In almost every case, once you get started and warmed up, you get into the movements, do all the reps, and go all the way. It's a little psychological game that you can play on yourself, and somehow it continues to work time after time. As it has been said, "just showing up is 90 percent of success," so just get those workout shoes and shorts on, get to a machine or a weight, and start out slowly. You'll warm up and keep going.

2. The solo mountain climber's focus and discipline.

When you are heading up the side of Yosemite's El Capitan, climbing without ropes or tools, there is no looking up or down, no thinking about what's coming or how hard it will be. The same applies to weightlifting when the only thing that matters is what you need to do at that moment: focus on the now. Another advantage of being in the moment while working out is the clearing of your mind, in a meditative way, so that all distractions are ignored. You will be calmer, and by paying close attention, your form and posture will be better, and you will be less likely to cause an injury.

3. The mirror, the scale, and the tape measure.

The numbers don't lie, exaggerate, or try to please your ego. They are the reality that will testify to the depth and duration of your commitment to building your body, getting your weight where it belongs, and getting that gut flatter. Start with a benchmark set of measurements, and check in every week. Look at yourself in the mirror without criticism or disappointment and just take notice of how your pecs (chest muscles) and abdominals look: a little soft, a layer of fat. Same for the arms and legs. Weigh yourself before breakfast, and write down the number each week, or daily if you prefer. Same for the tape measurement. Over time, you will see and record progress, and that will help solidify your commitment to your long-term objectives.

Inspirational Quotes

1. "Tough times don't last, but tough people do." — Richard Shuller (2020).

This quote applies to all aspects of life but has found special appreciation among professional lifters who push to their absolute limits. But especially for you as you are beginning weightlifting and conditioning, there are times when it isn't fun, like that last pull-up or barbell curl. Your thighs may be burning after three sets of squats or splits, and that last set of dumbbell rows may have you breathing pretty hard. But every time the set is over, and the rest begins, the pain and burning feeling subsides, and the workout always ends with a feeling of work well done, a sense of satisfaction. You are tough and getting tougher.

2. "To be a champion, you must act like a champion." — Lou Ferrigno (2020).

Lou Ferrigno, a champion weightlifter who played the Incredible Hulk, contributed to this recommended mindset because he believes that strength comes from within. A championship attitude is attainable by all of us if we believe in ourselves and envision the well-muscled, well-defined body we are working to achieve. But it goes further: If you want to become a well-built bodybuilder, you need to work out like one. Positive thinking is essential to motivate and inspire you, but without hard work and the determination to give it your all, positive thinking is just a dream.

3. "Don't wish it were easier. Wish you were better." — Jim Rohn (2020).

The thought leads us to expect that the workout, the lifting and pulling, the squatting and dipping, needs to be intensive, to challenge us. That leads to the realization that if it's easy, it's not being done right. You need to work to challenge your muscles to the point that muscle cells and fibers are damaged and need to self-repair through hypertrophy. The attitude that will carry you from passive to proactive is the recognition that it's a simple formula: strength is directly proportional to the effort that is invested in each workout. Of course, a hard workout can be followed in two days by a less intensive workout to aid recovery, but then be sure to make the next workout more intensive. It will pay off in the long-term.

4. "It never gets easier. You just get stronger." — Unknown (2020).

The idea is to add weights progressively when you can handle more without reducing reps, sets, or rest intervals. For example, head over to the dumbbell rack, and pick up a heavy weight you can do just one rep of a bicep curl or at most two. Do you wish you could do more reps? Find the weight you can lift or curl for eight reps and have the patience and confidence to know that in a reasonable time, with discipline, you will advance gradually from the lighter weight to the heavier ones and beyond. Just follow the basic practice of lifting weights that max out at eight to 10 reps, do the three sets, and be sure to rest between sets and between workouts.

5. "You have to be at your strongest when you're feeling at your weakest." — Unknown (2020).

This inspiration encourages weightlifters and cardio athletes to reach deep inside for the strength that they know is there. Imagine that you are a runner who is training for a marathon or other long-distance competition. The only time you can train is early in the morning before work, even in the cold and dark of winter. You need to roll out of bed at 5:30 a.m., wash your face, put on your running shoes, head outside, hit the road, and run into a biting cold headwind. What does it feel like to go through this, day after day, for months? This is what inner strength is all about, and it illustrates, in the extreme, what someone chooses to do to reach an objective. You probably will not have to work out under such an extreme condition. You'll be indoors, warm, lifting weights you can manage, and working to a reasonable, yet difficult peak of effort. But think of that runner in the dark, cold, early morning, and let it carry you to a better effort each day.

Chapter 10: Questions and Answers

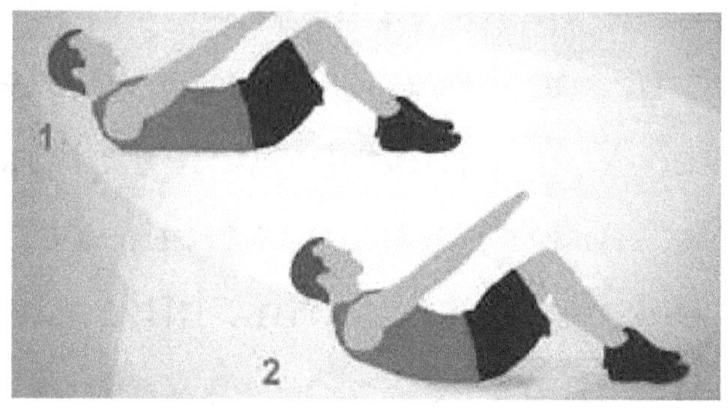

In order to stay fit the authors of the 7-Minute Workout suggest that you do this workout three times a week. The best time for you to do this workout is probably before or after breakfast, lunch or dinner. Even though you will only be performing circuits 2 and 3, it is suggested by the author that you consider doing circuit 1 too in order to warm up gradually.

The 7-Minute Workout for Seniors is a very beneficial workout routine for anyone. It is especially beneficial for people who are just beginning to exercise or individuals who have been diagnosed with heart disease, diabetes or osteoporosis. It is beneficial for people who are just beginning to exercise because it will help them become more fit and healthy. It is beneficial for people who have been diagnosed with heart disease, diabetes or osteoporosis because it can help reduce their risk of developing other diseases associated with sedentary lifestyles such as obesity or cardiovascular disease. This workout can also be used to improve muscle strength, balance and coordination. The 7-Minute Workout for Seniors is a great workout routine for individuals who are just beginning a fitness program or persons who want a simple and easy workout routine that helps them stay fit.

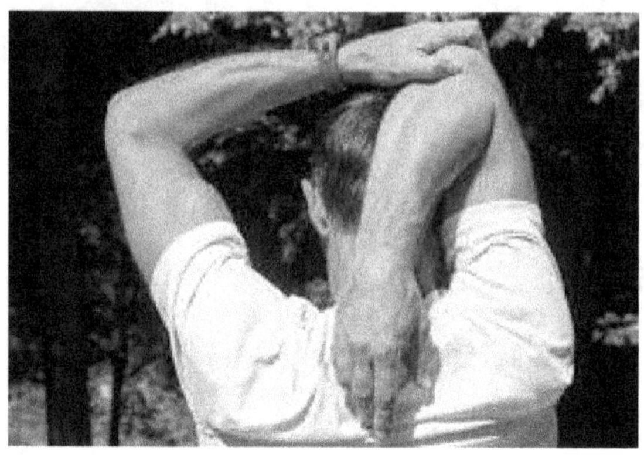

How to Improve Your Performance:

1) Always remember that you should warm up before doing any exercises.

2) The 7-Minute Workout for Seniors consists of four sets of exercises. For each set do 3 minutes (or 5 minutes in case you are doing circuit 2) with no rest in between the exercises.

3) The warm up should last about five minutes. It is recommended that you pick exercises that make your muscles feel a slight burning sensation and that also help you warm up slowly.

4) The 6 exercises consist of 1 minute, 2 minutes, 3 minutes and 4 minutes respectively. In order to learn more about how to do these exercises it is suggested by the author to check out the book titled "The 7-Minute Workout."

5) The cool down consists of three exercises and should last about two minutes.

6) You should drink plenty of water every day. At least one liter will be sufficient for the average person.

7) Eat a healthy diet to ensure adequate supplies of protein, carbohydrates and fats for your muscles. Also, eat plenty of different fruits and vegetables to ensure that you will get all the vitamins and minerals you need.

8) Plan to work out at different times in your week so you won't become bored or irritated by this workout routine. The book

also suggests that you find a friend with similar goals as you do to help motivate yourself to include a fitness routine in your life regularly.

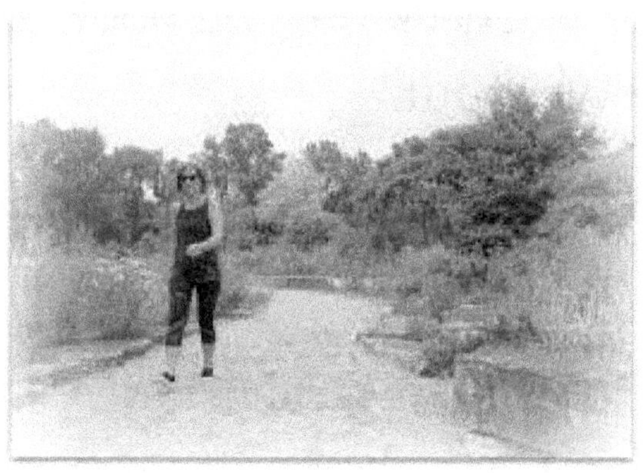

Questions and answers on the 7-minute workout for the seniors:

1. Can men do this workout?

This workout is be particularly beneficial for men. By doing this workout regularly the author of the book claims that it can help prevent heart disease and diabetes as well. This routine has also been proven to maintain muscle strength as we get older which is very important because it can improve balance and reduce the risk of falling which is one of the leading causes of death for seniors.

2. What are some other benefits of doing this workout?

This particular routine is good because it helps you improve your balance, coordination and bone density. It also helps you strengthen your cardiovascular fitness, muscles balance, coordination, bone density and muscle strength.

3. How many sets of exercises do I need to do?

The book suggests that you should do three sets of each exercise for about a minute. You also should perform each circuit three times before progressing to the next one. Progressing from one circuit to another by increasing your repetitions (e.g., three sets of 10 each exercise). The warm up should last about five minutes and you should work up to about 80 percent of your maximum heart rate and then decrease it in order to recover. It is also suggested that the cool down should last about 1-2 minutes. It is also important that you drink plenty of water throughout each day and eat a healthy diet in order for your muscles to recover faster.

4. Does the 7-Minute Workout for Seniors put a lot of pressure on my joints?

This workout routine is designed to be gentle for your joints because it is low impact and no knee or ankle weights are required.

5. How much space do I need to do this workout?

Since the 7-Minute Workout for Seniors consists of only three exercises that can be done at home or in other small places, it will not take up much space at all! It is very easy to do this workout routine.

6. What is the difference between circuit 1 and 2?

Circuit 1 consists of exercises that target your muscles and help them recover after performing other exercises. Circuit 2 consists of strength training exercises that target flexor and extensor muscles in order to improve your performance in activities such as walking, running, swimming or golfing.

7. Will I get bored doing this workout routine?

It is recommended by the author to use different times in your week for working out so you won't become bored. You may also want to find a friend with similar goals as you do to help motivate yourself.

The 7-Minute Workout for Seniors is a very beneficial workout routine for anyone. It is especially beneficial for people who are just beginning to exercise or individuals who have been diagnosed with heart disease, diabetes or osteoporosis. It is beneficial for people who are just beginning to exercise because it will help them become more fit and healthy. It is beneficial for people who have been diagnosed with heart disease, diabetes or osteoporosis because it can help reduce their risk of developing other diseases associated with sedentary lifestyles such as obesity or cardiovascular disease. This workout can also be used to improve muscle strength, balance and coordination. The 7-Minute Workout for Seniors is a great workout routine for individuals who are just beginning a fitness program or persons who want a simple and easy workout routine that helps them stay fit.

– This book will benefit you because it will help you improve your health by reducing your risk of developing many illnesses. The seven exercises contained in this book will help relax the muscles after a hard workout and also improve your cardiovascular fitness, balance, coordination, bone density and muscle strength.

– This workout is very beneficial because it does not take up much space at all! This routine consists of three sets of 6 exercises in order to be completed within seven minutes. It is very easy to do this workout routine. It can be done at home, the gym or even in a hotel room.

– This workout routine will help you improve your cardiovascular fitness because it contains exercises that target your muscles and help them recover after performing other exercises. Also, this routine helps relax the muscles after a hard workout and also improves your cardiovascular fitness, balance, coordination, bone density and muscle strength.

- This workout routine will help you stay fit because it can help prevent heart disease and diabetes. It can also develop your muscles strength as well.

- This routine helps improve muscle strength, balance and coordination. This workout also has been proven to maintain muscle strength as we get older which is very important because it can improve balance and reduce the risk of falling which is one of the leading causes of death for seniors.

- The 7-Minute Workout for Seniors consists of four sets of exercises that are all targeted for different parts of the body such as the chest, back, shoulders, arms, hips and thighs or legs. The warm up consists of three exercises in order to be completed within five minutes. The 6 exercises of this routine consist of 3 minutes, 4 minutes, 1 minute and 2 minutes respectively. In order to learn more about how to do these exercises it is suggested by the author to check out the book titled "The 7-Minute Workout."

– The cool down consists of three exercises and should last about two minutes.

– This workout routine has also been proven to maintain muscle strength as we get older which is very important because it can improve balance and reduce the risk of falling which is one of the leading causes of death for seniors.

– Information about why you should drink plenty of water everyday in order for your muscles to recover faster.

– Eat a healthy diet that provides you with adequate supplies of protein, carbohydrates and fats. Also eat plenty of different fruits and vegetables to ensure that you will get all the vitamins and minerals you need.

– Mix up your workout routine. Make sure that you plan to work out at different times in your week so you'll never get bored or irritated by this workout routine.

– You should drink plenty of water every day and eat a healthy diet in order for your muscles to recover faster.

Mediterranean Diet

This book portrays the dietary example regularly endorsed in investigations that recommend it's a sound method of eating.

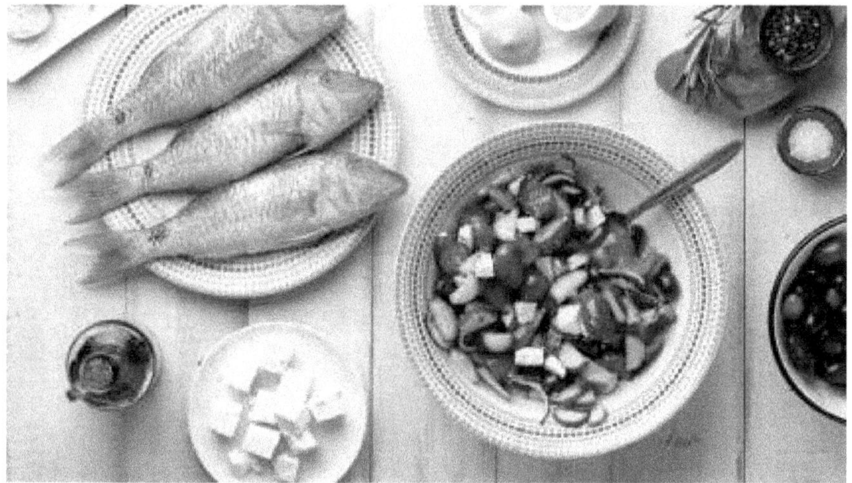

Table of Contents

Basics:

The Mediterranean eating routine depends on the customary food sources that individuals used to eat in nations like Italy and Greece back in 1960.

Analysts noticed that these individuals were uncommonly solid contrasted with Americans and had an okay of numerous way of life illnesses.

Various examinations have now shown that the Mediterranean eating routine can cause weight reduction and help forestall coronary episodes, strokes, type 2 diabetes and sudden passing.

There is nobody right approach to follow the Mediterranean eating routine, as there are numerous nations around the Mediterranean ocean and individuals in various regions may have eaten various food varieties.

Think about the entirety of this as an overall rule, not something written in stone. The arrangement can be changed in accordance with your individual requirements and inclinations.

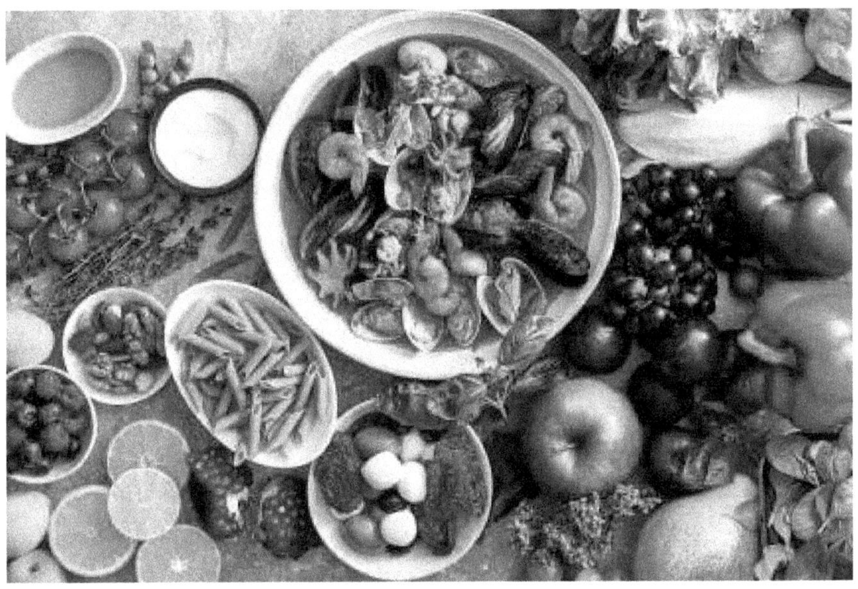

Historical and research overview:

Diets devoured by Mediterranean populaces have been a subject of revenue since relic, with later examinations zeroed in on their apparent medical advantages. Crafted by Ancel Keys during the 1950s set up the to a great extent plant-based Mediterranean eating routine as the first model for current dietary rules in the United States and somewhere else. As a social model for dietary improvement, the Mediterranean eating routine can be suggested for the two its medical advantages and its acceptability. Given overall patterns toward dietary consistency, exemplary Mediterranean eating regimens might be turning out to be imperiled species, and much fundamental and applied exploration is expected to characterize the manners by which such customary and invigorating dietary examples can be protected and advanced.

Abstract:

The Mediterranean practice offers a cousine wealthy in colors and aromas which support the taste and the soul of the individuals who live in agreement with nature. Everybody is discussing the Mediterranean eating routine, yet few are the individuals who do it appropriately, in this way producing a great deal of disarray in the peruser. Thus for some it agrees with the pizza, others recognized it with the noodles with meat sauce, in a combination of pseudo recorded customs and old stories that don't assist with settling the inquiry that is at the premise of any eating routine: consolidate and balance the food in order to fulfill the subjective and quantitative necessities of an individual and it could be said, jam his wellbeing using substances that assist the body with performing typical crucial capacities. The reason for our work is to exhibit that the mix of taste and wellbeing is an objective that can be totally completed by everyone, in spite of the individuals who accept that lone a liberal caloric admission can ensure the decency of a dish and the fulfillment of the buyers. That ought not be a flat out oddity, since the sound practices of the Mediterranean cooking we have utilized for quite a while in a wide assortment of delicious gastronomic decisions, from welcoming colors and solid aromas and totally in accordance with wellbeing.

History, territories and traditions:

The customary diets of nations lining the Mediterranean Sea contrast marginally so there are various variants of the Mediterranean diet. In any case, in 1993 the Harvard School of Public Health, Oldways Preservation and Exchange Trust, and the European Office of the World Health Organization presented the Mediterranean Diet Pyramid as a manual for help acclimate individuals with the most well-known foods of the district. A greater amount of an eating design than a stringently controlled diet plan, the pyramid stressed certain foods dependent on the dietary practices of Crete, Greece, and southern Italy during the mid-twentieth century. Around then, these nations showed low paces of ongoing illness and higher than normal grown-up future in spite of having restricted admittance to medical services. It was accepted that the diet—principally foods grown from the ground, beans, nuts, entire grains, fish, olive oil, limited quantities of dairy, and red wine—added to their medical advantages. The pyramid likewise featured day by day exercise and the gainful social parts of eating dinners together.

The Mediterranean diet is an essentially plant-based eating plan that incorporates day by day admission of entire grains, olive oil, organic products, vegetables, beans and different vegetables, nuts, spices, and flavors. Different foods like animal proteins are eaten in more modest amounts, with the favored animal protein being fish and seafood.

The Mediterranean eating regimen has it's anything but a bit of land thought about exceptional in its sort, the Mediterranean bowl, which antiquarians call "the cradle of society", on the grounds that inside its topographical boundaries the entire history of the antiquated world occurred.

At its banks extended the valley of the Nile, the site of an old and progressed human advancement, and the two extraordinary bowls of the Tigris and Euphrates, which were the climate of the development of the Sumerians, Assyrians, Babylonians and Persians. In the Mediterranean district emerged the force of the Cretans, then, at that point arose the Phoenicians and the learned Greeks up to the arising force of Rome, which permitted the domain to turn into the "great land" between the East and the West. From that time, the Mediterranean turned into the gathering spot of individuals who, with their contacts, have every now and then altered societies, customs, dialects, religions and perspectives about changing constantly way of life with the advancement of history. The conflict of these two societies delivered their fractional reconciliation so even the dietary patterns converged to some extent.

The beginnings of the "Mediterranean Diet" are lost in time since they sink into the dietary patterns of the Middle Ages, in which the antiquated Roman custom - on the model of the Greek - recognized in bread, wine and oil items an image of rustic culture and rural (and images chose of the new confidence), enhanced by sheep cheddar, vegetables (leeks, mallow, lettuce, chicory, mushrooms), little meat and a solid inclination for fish and seafood (of which old Rome was ravenous. The rich classes adored the new fish (who ate for the most part singed in olive oil or barbecued) and seafood, particularly shellfish, eating crude or seared. Captives of Rome, be that as it may, was ordained helpless food comprises of bread and a large portion of a pound of olives and olive oil a month, with some salted fish, once in a while a little meat. The Roman practice before long conflicted with the style of food imported from the way of life of the Germanic people groups, predominantly migrants, living in close congruity with the backwoods, gotten from something similar, with chasing, cultivating and assembling, the vast majority of the food assets. Raised pigs of fat, generally utilized in the kitchen, and developed vegetables in little gardens near the camps. The couple of grains developed were not used to make bread, yet lager. The conflict of these two societies delivered their fractional coordination so even the dietary patterns converged to some degree. In any case, the Roman culture showed itself reluctant to change the style of "Mediterranean" of taking care of with that boorish. The critical components of the Mediterranean diet, which is the group of three oil bread and wine, were sent out rather in areas of mainland Europe by the devout orders, which moved in those districts to proselytize those people groups. Bread, oil and wine, were truth be told the focal components of the Christian sacrament, yet they were subsequently received additionally in the taking care of the commoners of Europe. The new food culture brought into the world from the association and the combination between dietary examples of two distinct civilizations, the Christian Roman Empire and the Germanic, crossed with the progression of time with a third practice or that of the Arab world, which had fostered its own remarkable food culture on the southern shores of the Mediterranean.

Just Muslims gave a lift to a restoration of horticulture that affected the food model with the presentation of plant species known or utilized exclusively by the more affluent social classes, due to the exorbitant costs, for example, sugar stick, rice, citrus, eggplant, spinach and flavors, just as discovered use in the cooking of southern Europe, rose water, oranges, lemons, almonds and pomegranates. Islamic culture, hence, takes an interest in the change and change of the social solidarity of the Mediterranean, which Rome had constructed, and gives a definitive commitment to the new culinary model that was framing. Countless foods, passed by Muslims on Latin, drag their readiness procedures and plans.

Another occasion of incredible chronicled sway was, as it is notable, the disclosure of America by Europeans. This disclosure is likewise reflected in a "buy" with respect to the culinary practice of new foodstuffs like potatoes, tomatoes, corn, peppers and stew, just as various assortments of beans. The tomato, "colorful interest", decorative organic product just behind schedule thought about eatable, was the primary red vegetable that improved our crate of plants and later turned into an image of the Mediterranean cooking. On the off chance that the centrality of vegetables is quite possibly the most unique characters of the Mediterranean practice, it is essential to recollect the job of grains as the premise of straightforward cooking and as a weapon of day by day endurance, due to their "capacity to fill" lessening food cravings of helpless classes. The kind of cereals burned-through, just as the methods of change, accepts various aspects relying upon the topographical implications and customs that describe the populaces of the nations verging on the Mediterranean. Bread, polenta, couscous, soups, paella and pasta are various approaches to devour cereals.

This authentic way depicted permits distinguishing numerous similitudes between the Mediterranean diet and current diet of our precursors to show the presence of a genuine way that from the taking care of the Egyptians to the disclosure of America prompted the presentation of new foods, giving us the Mediterranean diet as we probably are aware today.

The Mediterranean diet, referred to fundamentally as a food model, upgrades the quality and wellbeing of foods and their connection to the place where there is beginning. It's anything but a straightforward cooking, however wealthy in creative mind and tastes, exploiting all parts of a sound diet. It's anything but a moral decision that safeguards the practices and customs of the people groups of the Mediterranean Basin. Taking care of can significantly influence the soundness of people; this is on the grounds that a decent dietary status assists with keeping a decent degree of wellbeing and anticipation of metabolic infections like heftiness, diabetes, hypertension, and so forth The Mediterranean Diet is likewise an asset for practical improvement is vital for every one of the nations verging on the Mediterranean, to the monetary and culture impact the food covers all through the district and the capacity to rouse a feeling of congruity and character for neighborhood individuals.

Eating behaviors and lifestyles:

The revelation of the medical advantages of the Mediterranean Diet is ascribed to the American researcher Ancel Keys of the University of Minnesota School of Power, which called attention to the relationship between's cardiovascular illness and diet interestingly. Ancel Keys, in the fifties, was struck by a marvel, which proved unable, from the start, give a full clarification. The helpless populace of unassuming communities of southern Italy was, against all forecasts, a lot more grounded than the affluent residents of New York, both of their own family members who emigrated in before a very long time in the United States. Keys proposed that this relied upon food, and attempted to approve his unique knowledge, concentrating on foods that made up the diet of these populaces. In this manner, he drove the celebrated "Seven Countries Study" (directed in Finland, Holland, Italy, United States, Greece, Japan and Yugoslavia), to report the connection between ways of life, sustenance and cardiovascular infection between various populaces, including through cross-sectional examinations, having the option to demonstrate logically the dietary benefit of the Mediterranean diet and its commitment to the strength of the populaces that embraced it.

From this examination arose obviously, as the populaces that had embraced a diet dependent on the Mediterranean Diet introduced an extremely low pace of cholesterol in the blood and, thus, a base level of coronary illness. This was mostly because of the copious utilization of olive oil, bread, pasta, vegetables, spices, garlic, red onions, and different foods of vegetable beginning contrasted with a fairly moderate utilization of meat.

The American nutritionist portrayed the Mediterranean diet thusly: "... hand crafted minestrone, pasta, all things considered, with pureed tomatoes and a sprinkling of Parmesan, just sporadically improved with a couple of bits of meat or presented with a little fish of the spot beans and macaroni ..., such a lot of bread, never eliminated from the broiler in excess of a couple of hours prior to being eaten, and nothing with which spread it, heaps of new vegetables sprinkled with olive oil, a little part of meat or fish several times each week and in every case new organic product for dessert"

In any case, we should bring up that the Mediterranean diet can't deliver, without anyone else, the advantages recorded above in the event that you don't change simultaneously other danger factors (clearly those modifiable). Truth be told, ischemic coronary illness depends not just on mistakes in the sythesis of the diet, to which joins a predominant job, yet in addition by different variables, like a decreased or missing actual work, caloric admission in abundance of the energy needs of the organic entity, the presence of metabolic sicknesses like diabetes and weight, stress, cigarette smoking, undeniable degrees of homocysteine in the blood, significant degrees of fatty substances. In this way, it's anything but amazing that about portion of all instances of stroke happen in people with an ordinary degree of cholesterol in the blood. To forestall a coronary failure is along these lines basic to take not just a reasonable diet (as is undoubtedly the Mediterranean diet), yet in addition a solid way of life (as Ancel Keys had effectively called attention to).

In 2007, an examination led by the National Institutes of Health showed that moderate active work is related with an abatement in mortality from cardiovascular infection.

Indeed, active work assists with lessening some danger factors for cardiovascular illness like hypertension, insulin opposition, hypertriglyceridemia, low HDL and the presence of stoutness. Besides, practice coupled to appropriate sustenance can diminish the blood levels of LDL. Different advantages incorporate the beginning of atherosclerosis, since practice improves myocardial capacity, expands the vasodilator limit, muscle tone, and decreases fiery pressure.

You may ask why you have spent such countless words, for a very long time or somewhere in the vicinity, to upgrade a diet that needn't bother with any presentation. The explanation is that the pattern away from the conventional diet for food designs commonplace of the princely society has been continuous for a long time. The Mediterranean Diet is subsequently portrayed by the fair utilization of foods wealthy in fiber, cancer prevention agents and unsaturated fats, a solid methodology intended to lessen the utilization of creature fats and cholesterol in a diet with a fitting harmony between energy admission and consumption. The connections between the macronutrient energy answer to those perceived as sufficient, i.e 55–60% of carbs of which 80% complex carbs (bread, pasta, rice), 10–15% of proteins about 60% of creature beginning (particularly white meat, fish), 25–30%

fat (for the most part Olive Oil). The rules created by nutritionists to improve the dietary patterns of buyers can be addressed by a compelling picture, the "Food Pyramid" intended without precedent for 1992 by the U.S. Division of Agriculture, which basically addresses a reasonable and adjusted method of eating, showing the extents and the frequencies with which foods ought to be devoured, style that corresponds with the Mediterranean Model distinguished by the physiologist Ancel Keys.

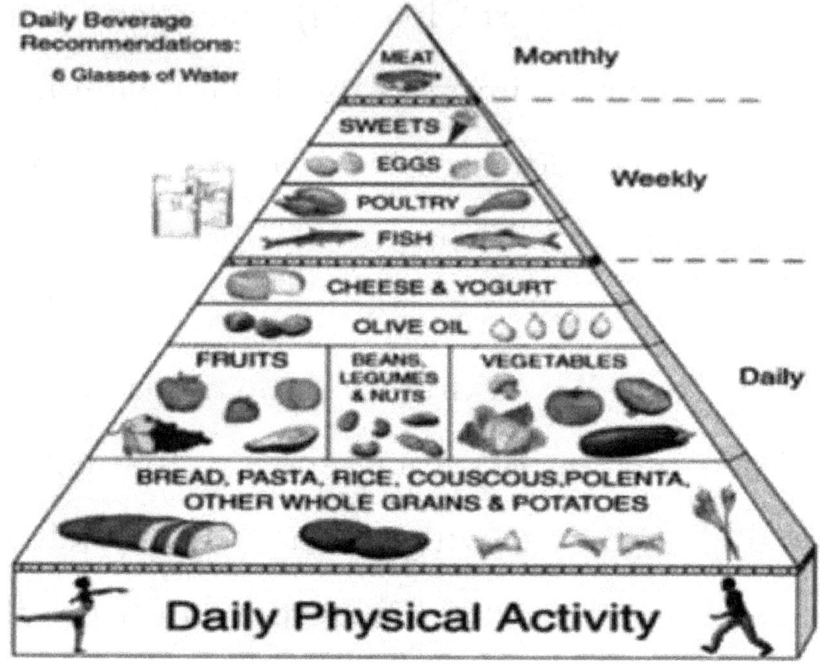

The primary ideas of the Food Pyramid are the "Proportionality", that is the perfect measure of foods to look over for each gathering, the "partition" standard amount of food in grams, which is expected as the unit of estimation to be a decent taking care of, the "assortment", i.e., the significance of changing the decisions inside a food gathering, and "balance" in the utilization of specific foods, like fat or desserts. As should be obvious, at the foundation of the pyramid are grains, trailed by foods grown from the ground, vegetables, olive oil, low-fat cheddar and yogurt, which ought to be eaten every day. Meat isn't prohibited, yet is given the inclination to that of chicken, hare and turkey than hamburger. Alongside fish and eggs ought to be eaten a couple of times each week, for the stock of top notch protein. Hamburger or red meat ought to be eaten a couple of times each month.

Each gathering incorporates foods, which are significantly "same" on the wholesome arrangement, as in they give almost similar kind of supplements. Clearly, inside a similar gathering, foods in spite of being homogeneous with one another can have little contrasts as far as quality and amount of patrimony in supplements. In any case, this doesn't influence the idea of "compatibility" of foods. The last truth be told, in the event that they have a place with a similar gathering, being healthfully same, might be substitutes for one another, without, in any case, influencing the sufficiency of the diet, furnished you follow the assortment. In nature doesn't exist a "total" food, for example it contains every one of the supplements the body needs, and that is the reason it is important to fluctuate however much as could be expected food decisions and appropriately join foods from the various gatherings. An exceptionally fluctuated Diet not just stays away from the danger of nourishing lopsided characteristics and conceivable subsequent metabolic awkward nature, however it additionally fulfills the flavor of battling the dullness of flavors. Each gathering expected is addressed by at any rate a bit of the foods that establish it, to shift the decisions inside a similar group.The idea of sum is utilized to point our consideration on: • Portion of food, as amount in grams, which is viable with the prosperity of our body, so there are nothing but bad foods or terrible, yet their impact relies upon the sum devoured day by day, the decision of a suitable number of parts of food should cover all the food bunches in the pyramid every day to make certain to take every one of the supplements; actual work, not to fall into an inactive way of life, the WQ of reference is a brief stroll at a lively speed, we suggest at any rate 2 WQ/day which is 30 minutes walk likewise detachable during the day. The QB of food and development, if appropriately adjusted to the requirements of the individual, permit arranging the ways of life towards a harmony between food admission and energy use. Along these lines, you can stay away from the overweight and battling weight that inclines the life form to an expanded danger of metabolic illnesses (diabetes, hypertension, and so forth), cardiovascular sicknesses and even malignancy.

Cereals:

The main group, the oats and tubers, incorporates bread, pasta, rice, corn, oats, grain, spelled and potatoes. This group should be available in consistently taking care of (ideally with entire foods since more fiber-rich) and in a few parts, in light of the fact that these foods are the main wellspring of starch, effectively usable energy from our body. This doesn't imply that grains ought to be eaten in over the top amount, yet to be burned-through with respect to their requirements. It is adequate to say, via model, 120g of uncooked pasta gives 427 calories, 80g is identical to 285 calories to and 55g to 196 calories. Additionally, a portion of these foods contain nutrients of the B bunch and a decent lot of protein (as in they come up short on some fundamental amino acids in adequate amounts, among which, especially lysine) that, related with vegetables, comprise a supper with a high protein admission and high natural worth, practically identical to meat. This mix happens habitually in our diet since the cereals and their subsidiaries are the fundamental elements for the planning of numerous dishes. The most popular models are the principal dishes from grains and vegetables: these dishes, because of the ability of proteins of the oats to be "integral" to the proteins found in vegetables, and giving commonly the amino acids of which are uniquely missing (separately lysine for cereals and methionine for vegetables), understand an improvement of the nature of the two proteins, which all in all gets like that of meat proteins.

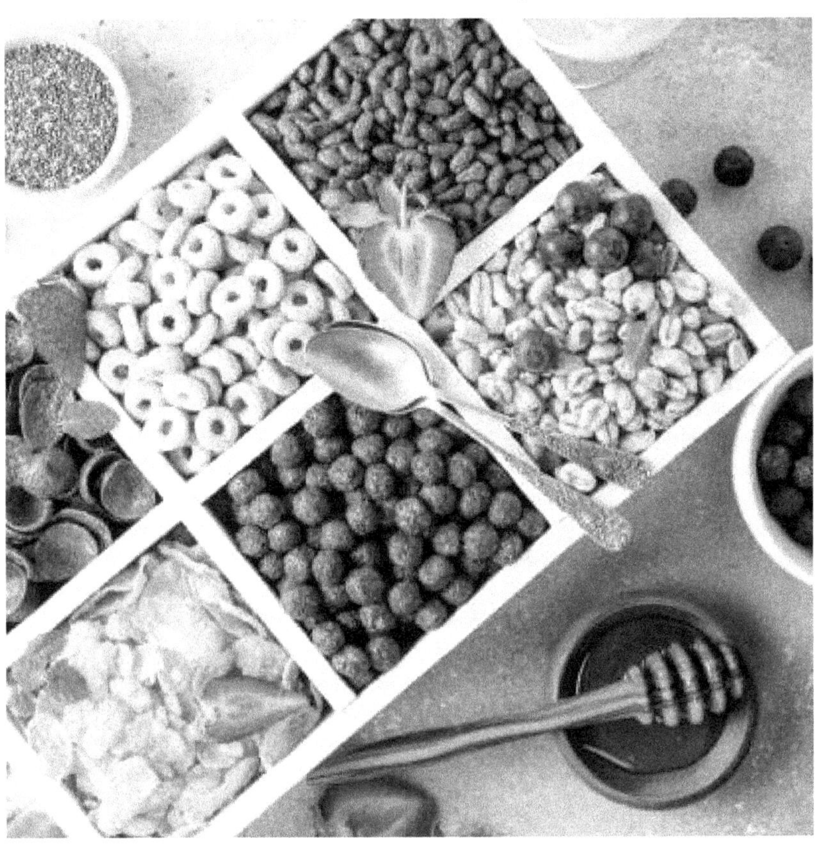

Fruits and vegetables:

The group of products of the soil likewise incorporates fresh vegetables like green beans. They should be stringently occasional and as new as could really be expected: just along these lines, they can foster better their quality and are more delicious on the grounds that aged to the warmth of the sun.

Vegetables and natural products aged in nursery, in any case, require a more prominent stock of pesticides and not exploiting the warmth of the sun, they are less plentiful in nutrients and supplements. Foods grown from the ground are a significant wellspring of fiber, Vitamin A (discovered fundamentally in tomatoes, peppers, carrots, melon, apricots, and so on), Vitamin C (basically in tomatoes, strawberries, citrus organic products, kiwi, and so on), different nutrients and numerous minerals, similar to potassium. Furthermore, foods grown from the ground contain these minor parts (cancer prevention agents and others), which play a significant defensive activity for the body and water that can reach even 95% of the weight (watermelon). Besides, contain any important amounts of dietary fiber (cellulose, hemicellulose and gelatin), which in spite of having a characteristic healthy benefit, has a part in working with the intestinal travel and in directing the degrees of blood cholesterol and glucose More reliable is, all things considered, the commitment in sugar (sucrose and fructose) produced using natural product. It is fundamental that foods in this group are available consistently and a lot in nourishment.

The part of foods grown from the ground in the diet is likewise connected to its physiological controller of water balance for their significant inventory of water. Besides, the substance of potassium salts can balance the acids emerging from a taking care of today again and again wealthy in creature proteins. At long last, we ought not fail to remember the job of these foods in the counteraction of weight, because of their high substance of fiber and water and low in calories that give (12 calories for zucchini, 16 calories for eggplant, 14Kcal for cucumbers, 12 Kcal for fennel, etc) contrasted with the volume ingested and the high satisfying force.

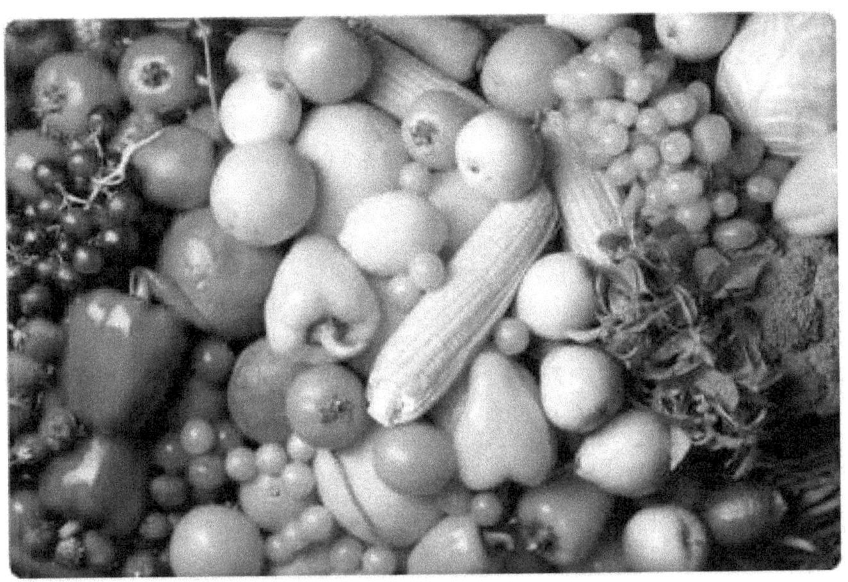

Milk and dairy products:

The dairy group incorporates milk, yogurt, cheddar and dairy items. This food group gives calcium in an exceptionally bioavailable structure, that is effectively acclimatized by the body. Also, these foods contain high natural quality proteins and a few nutrients (B2 and A). Inside the group are favored low-fat milk, dairy items and low-fat cheddar. The calcium in milk (either be in part or totally skimmed) and its subordinates is the main supplement, with the idiosyncrasy to be better assimilated and utilized by the body. The milk contains more than 1g of calcium per liter, while cheddar, as per the innovation of readiness, contains a few more percent, so that in the hard cheeses and prepared the amount of calcium can be multiple times higher than that present in milk to approach weight. Notwithstanding calcium, these foods give huge measures of proteins of high organic worth; among these casein is the most addressed (the part that coagulates when the milk sours and which frames the reason for the readiness of cheddar) and lactalbumin which together comprise 3.5%. The utilization of milk is in this way the most prompt manner to make the supplements normal for the group, however a similarly substantial option is addressed by yogurt and cheeses, where they exist instances of lactose bigotry, because of the need or nonattendance of an intestinal catalyst called "lactase", liable for the breakdown of lactose in the two mixtures galactose and glucose.

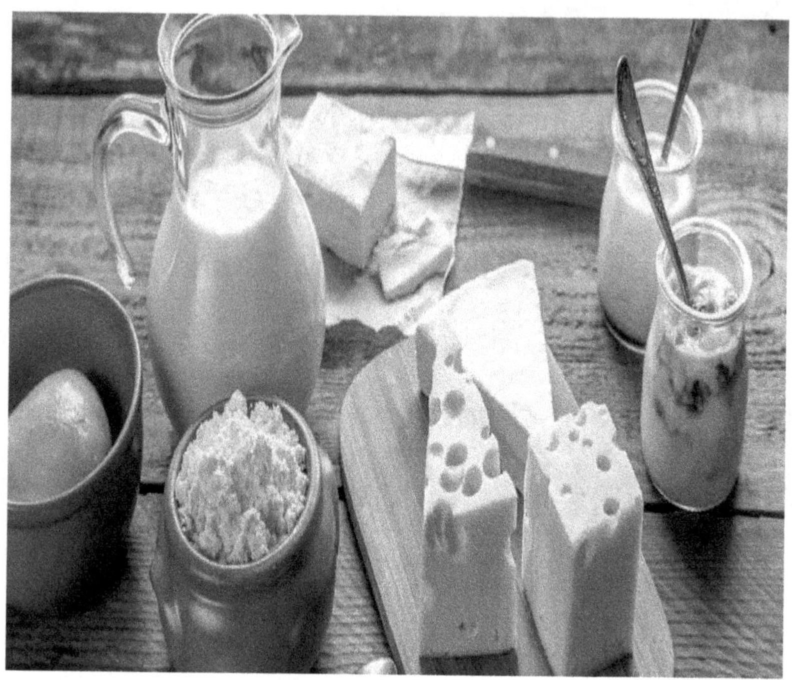

Meat, eggs and fish:

The meat is viewed as a food indispensable by ideals of its high protein content (from 15 to 25%) and of high natural worth, ready to make every one of the amino acids important for protein blend (fundamental amino acids) in ideal sums. It additionally gives B-complex nutrients and minor components, especially iron, zinc and copper. Notwithstanding, be careful not all foods in this group are something similar: between the meats is smarter to favor those lean both cow-like and pork, and white meat and fish and better moderate the utilization of fatter meat and more wieners. For eggs in sound subjects is permitted a utilization of egg 2–3 times each week. Foods in this group should be available in our diet a couple of times each week, except for red meat, which ought to be eaten a couple of times each month. Any food of creature beginning having a place with this group, regardless of whether new, chilled and frozen, gives protein of high natural worth, minor components and nutrients of the B complex, remembering for specific thiamine (nutrient B1), niacin (nutrient PP) and nutrient B12, the last is brought as a rule of foods of creature beginning. A few foods of this group additionally give non-insignificant amounts of different minerals, like iodine (in fish) and fat-dissolvable nutrients (nutrient An and D, contained basically in the liver).

The measure of protein contained in the food group is equivalent to 18–20% of the absolute weight, with higher qualities for saved meats (salami), where it might reach up to 37% because of the deficiency of water subsequent to drying.

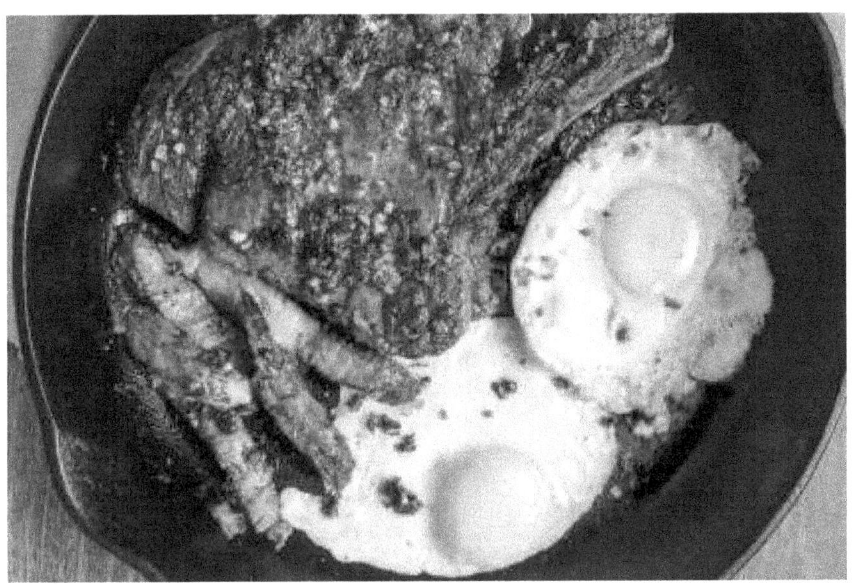

Dressing fats:

The dressing fats group incorporates vegetable fats, like olive oil (liked) and those of creature beginning: margarine, cream, bacon-fat and fat. Dressing fats improve the flavors and give fundamental unsaturated fats to the assimilation of fat-dissolvable nutrients, for the arrangement of the cell film and of some primary components of the cell. Notwithstanding, their utilization, particularly on account of creature fats, should be restricted for two reasons: they give numerous calories and, utilized in overabundance, address a danger factor for the beginning of corpulence, cardiovascular infections and tumors. There is an unmistakable connection between the utilization of soaked unsaturated fats and the beginning of Coronary Heart Disease and is subsequently not prescribed to supplant immersed fats with polyunsaturated. Olive oil is a critical component in the Mediterranean diet as it assists with forestalling cardiovascular infection. The phenols found in olive oil are undoubtedly amazing cancer prevention agents with calming and hostile to thrombotic, and some monounsaturated unsaturated fats found in olive oil are defensive for cardiovascular infection. Hence, the olive oil is generally alluded to as "sweeper of arteries".

Tips and tricks to get started:

- Breakfast ideas: Natural greek yogurt with local honey, berries and seeds, avocado whole wheat toast with olive oil, homemade smoothie with organic fruits

- Lunch ideas: Head to a salad bar and add avocado or wild fish as your protein, whole grain veggie sandwich with hummus, whole grain bowl (try quinoa or barley) with raw vegetables

- Snack ideas: Go nuts! Try dried fruits, nuts and seeds, snack on smoked salmon, eat raw fruit or vegetables and go for berries

- Dinner ideas: Mediterranean pizza with whole wheat dough, vegetables and cheese, grilled chicken with kale salad and grilled fish whole wheat tacos and avocado

Proven benefits:

Researchers have seriously examined the eating designs normal for the Mediterranean Diet for the greater part a century.

Soon after World War II, Ancel Keys and partners (counting Paul Dudley White, later President Eisenhower's heart specialist) coordinated the striking Seven Countries Study to look at the speculation that Mediterranean-eating designs contributed straightforwardly to improved wellbeing results. This long-running investigation inspected the wellbeing of just about thirteen thousand moderately aged men in the United States, Japan, Italy, Greece, the Netherlands, Finland, and afterward Yugoslavia.

At the point when the information were inspected, plainly individuals who ate a diet where foods grown from the ground, grains, beans, and fish were the premise of every day dinners were best. Beating the outline were inhabitants of Crete. Even after the hardships of World War II – and partially, maybe, as a result of them – the cardiovascular wellbeing of Crete inhabitants surpassed that of US occupants. Specialists ascribed the differences to diet.

Out of this broad work came an agreement that specific Mediterranean-eating designs were amazingly associated with great wellbeing. From this end arose the idea of a "Mediterranean Diet" that could advance deep rooted great wellbeing.

In ensuing years, hundreds if not large number of extra examinations have added to the collection of scientific proof supporting the "highest quality level" status of conventional Mediterranean Diet eating designs. These examinations show that eating the Med way may:

Extend your life

Improve cerebrum work

Safeguard you from constant sicknesses

Battle certain malignant growths

Lower your danger for coronary illness, hypertension and raised "awful" cholesterol levels

Shield you from diabetes

Help your weight reduction and the board efforts

Ward off despondency

Defend you from Alzheimer's infection

Ward off Parkinson's infection

Improve rheumatoid joint pain

Improve eye wellbeing

Decrease hazard of dental illness

Assist you with relaxing

Lead to better infants

Lead to improved fertility

Conclusion:

All in all, it very well may be said that the Mediterranean diet isn't just a monstrous abundance of foods and plans, yet in addition a significant resource among individuals and domain: the people groups of the Mediterranean have consistently found in their property their lives, and are brought into the world from the dirt the vast majority of the results of the diet. The relentless assortment of items in the grounds of the Mediterranean need to guarantee, whenever devoured in a fitting way, all that our body requires to work. Today taking care of has become a significant perspective in the existence of each person. The specialty of eating great has gotten a model for people in general to follow, but on the other hand are expanding non-autochthonous ways of life, which are in some objective populace a prolific ground to build the quantity of adepts of these new ways. In the clinical field the diet has gotten perhaps the main viewpoints to be observed at all phases of the existence of the subject: the counteraction of numerous illnesses to diet treatment that discovers increasingly more acknowledgment among doctors and patients. The achievement of the Mediterranean diet is it's anything but: a fluctuated diet portrayed by an intense usage of vegetables, natural products, grains, vegetables, fish, eggs, alongside a moderate admission of meat, oil and wine. A diet wealthy in custom and in relationship with one dynamic way of life is the model that everybody ought to follow.

CPSIA information can be obtained
at www.ICGtesting.com
Printed in the USA
LVHW010709020821
694270LV00012B/1200